THE DOCTOR BOOK

A Nuts And Bolts Guide To Patient Power

THE DOCTOR BOOK

A Nuts And Bolts Guide To Patient Power

by Wesley J. Smith
Illustrated by Stephanie O'Shaughnessy
Special medical consultant—Dr. Daniel V. Ehrensaft, M.D.

PRICE STERN SLOAN
Los Angeles

For Dad,
The song may be over,
but the melody lingers on . . .

Published by Price Stern Sloan, Inc.

ISBN: 0-89586-747-8

Acknowledgements

This book could not have been possible without the wholehearted cooperation of the following physicians whose intense dedication to healing I hope can be read between the lines: my special medical consultant Daniel V. Ehrensaft, M.D., whose energy and dedication opened so many doors and inspired so many ideas; Jerald S. Davitz, M.D.; Victor Berman, M.D.; Robert Fitzgerald, M.D.; Stephen L. Herr, M.D.; Mary Grace Horning, M.D.; Vicki Georges Hufnagel, M.D.; Michael Kamiel, M.D.; Charles E. Keenan, M.D.; E. Gaylon McCullough, M.D.; Glenn Pasternack, M.D., F.A.C.S.; Rebecca Plumer, M.D.; Samuel O. Sapin, M.D.; Tamar Singer, M.D.; Mark S. Van Houten, M.D.

Thanks also to the following persons and organizations, who provided invaluable assistance: Ruth Ancheta, A.A.H.C.C.; Ira Bates, Ph.D.; U.S. Congressman Anthony C. Beilensen; David Berglund, Attorney at Law; Salee Berman, M.A., C.N.M.; Gary Bess, M.S.W.; Bruce Bratton; Paula Carroll; Karen Davis; John V. Fenton; Linda Fishman; Howard O. Flushman; Arlene F. Flom; Stephen Gottschalk; Harold Greenberg, Attorney at Law; Paula H. Jolly; Nancy Kraemer; Kurt Hegetschweiler, D.C.; Mike Henbery, R.N., M.I.C.N.; Carol Kinsey; Steven Kozel, Phar. D.; Paul Lehman; Lowell Levin; Howard Lewis; Barbara Lopez; Alan Mann; Howard P. Marshall, D.P.M., M.S.Ed.; Ralph Nader; A.N. Norman, M.P.A.; Jack A. Rameson III, Attorney at Law; Jim Rodgers; Harvey Rosenfield; Janice Seib; Harrison W. Sommer; Lora B. Sanders; Mark Stuart, A.M.A.; Nathan A. Talbot; Nancy Tamarisk, R.N.; Ron Tamarisk, R.N.; Donna F. Ver Steeg, R.N., Ph.D., F.A.A.N.; Ken Wagstaff; Sam Yee; David I. Zeitlin.

American Academy of Facial, Plastic & Reconstructive Surgery; American Academy of Physicians; American Academy of Pediatrics; American Board of Emergency Medicine; American Board of Internal Medicine; American Chiropractic Association; American College of Surgeons; American Diabetes Association; American Heart Association; American Lung Association; American Medical Association; American Society of Anesthesiology; American Society of Cataract & Refractive Surgery; Arthritis Foundation; Association of American Medical Colleges; Blue Cross-Blue Shield of California; Brotman Medical Center; CIGNA Health Plan; California Board of Medical Quality Assurance; California Chiropractic Association; Centers for Disease Control; College of Osteopathic Medicine of the Pacific; Consumers for Medical Quality Incorporated; Council of Teaching Hospitals of the Association of

American Medical Colleges; Cystic Fibrosis Association; Epilepsy Foundation of America; FDA Drug Hotline; Family Service of America; Health Insurance Association of America; Joint Commission on Accreditation of Hospitals; Kaiser Permanente; Los Angeles County Medical Association; Los Angeles Free Clinic; Mayo Clinic; Medic Alert Foundation International; National Hospice Organization; Northridge Hospital; People's Medical Society; Public Citizen; The Bills Project; The First Church of Christ Scientist; The Risk Management Foundation; U.S. Department of Health & Human Services; United Way; The Veterans Administration.

And last, but not least, thanks to those friends, loved ones and associates whose support and enthusiasm has meant so much: my mother Leona Smith, Gladys Yarborough, Jennie Frankle-Ehrensaft, Davy Frankle, Diane and Bill Robison, Carla Mancari, Lorraine Sinkler, Adele Tinning, Shirley Strick, Gina Francis, Don Sterling, Guy Stockwell, John Albert, Linda Day, Lisa Marsoli, Nick Clemente, Leonard Stern, Ron Gold, Gloria Blackman, everyone at Price Stern Sloan and Terrie Frankle-Smith, my super-charged wife.

Table of Contents

Foreword

There is an old saying, "knowledge is power," which when you think about it makes a lot of sense. Without knowledge there can be no intelligent exercise of choice and without choice there is no freedom. And a person who is not free, by definition, has no power.

There are few areas in life where we need "knowledge power" as much as we do in health care. After all, it is the quality, and sometimes the length, of our lives and the lives of those we love that may be at stake every time we consult a doctor or accept treatment for a medical malady. With so much riding on the decisions we make, we need to have information—information which is accurate and complete enough to allow us to make intelligent choices about our own health care and that of our families, based on the facts, not myths or fear. In other words, "patient power" means being in control of our own health care.

Such patient power is essential, for in medicine as in life, it is what you *don't* know that really can, and too often does, hurt you—as it did my father.

Dad was one of those men who seemed indestructible—he had managed to survive the horrors of World War II, having come home from the Pacific Campaign with a battlefield commission, a chest full of medals and a bad case of malaria. From then on, he was never sick a day in life (as they say), until 1980, when he simply stopped feeling well.

It wasn't that Dad was sick, exactly, it's just that his sense of well-being left him and he began to exhibit a few of the symptoms that I now know are found in the American Cancer Society's "Seven Warning Signals" of cancer. Dad was concerned enough to get a "complete" physical, which he did in the summer of 1980. Unfortunately, Dad was not given a standard test which would, in all likelihood, have revealed the tumor that was growing inside him. That was the medical clinic's fault. It was Dad's fault that he didn't know enough to know that something had been left out and didn't think to ask.

By early 1981, my father's condition slowly deteriorated to the point that I became increasingly concerned for his health. When I would ask him if he was feeling well, he would say, "My doctor has given me a clean bill of health, and I trust him. All right, son?"

"All right, Dad." That answer was my mistake.

On Father's Day 1981, I received the shock of my life. In the eight weeks since I had last visited my father he had lost at least thirty pounds. Now, I wasn't just concerned, I was horrified! Dad's little white lie that he was on a diet didn't reduce the deep concern my mother and I felt, and we again badgered him into getting a physical. This time the test which had been omitted the previous year, a sigmoidoscopy by proctoscope, *was given* and the cancer in my father's colon was discovered—but too late. The disease had already begun its deadly march through my father's body. He died on February 12, 1984.

I am convinced that my father's disease could and should have been diagnosed one year before it finally was. I also believe that the responsibility for that omission is, at least in part, my father's own, because he blindly accepted what a doctor told him instead of listening to what his own body was screaming—a message which might have made the difference between life and a posthumous book dedication.

In the motion picture *Annie Hall,* Woody Allen's character says that one of the pleasures of being a writer is that you can rewrite history and give it a better ending. Here is my rewrite of 1981:

Dad has a primary care physician, Caring N. Thorough, M.D., who has been his doctor for several years. Dr. Thorough knows my father and his health intimately, and perhaps more importantly he possesses a detailed knowledge of my father's medical history, which includes the facts that his mother and two siblings had cancer, and that he was exposed to radiation during the atomic bomb tests in Nevada in the early fifties. This background information keeps Dr. Thorough ever-watchful for the early signs of cancer in my father. The doctor would insist that Dad undergo a complete physical annually, and would include in that physical an examination by proctoscope. The exam of 1980 would then uncover Dad's condition and he would live to tell the tale.

Or, another scenario: My father has educated himself about the warning signs of cancer and believes that his body may be telling him something. And, even though he receives his medical care through a governmentally funded clinic, he does not allow himself to be just another face in the crowd. During the examination he asks the doctor conducting the physical, "Are there any tests beyond this examination that I could take to make sure that your diagnosis of hemorrhoids is telling the whole story?" The doctor would then tell him about the proctoscope, Dad would insist on receiving the test and the cancer would be discovered.

But what *did* happen to my father has taught me that it is each individual's responsibility to nurture his or her body, keep it properly maintained and have it repaired when problems do arise. Health care professionals have undergone years of education, training and experience so that they may assist us in this task, *not do it for us.* We are the ones who must bear the final responsibility for our own health care since we are the ones who will have to live with the consequences of it.

And so, what I am advocating is a team effort based on mutual respect, honesty and equality, in which you and your physician (or health insurance agent or nurse or other health care professional) work together to make intelligent choices, all of which are aimed at maximizing the quality of your life, your health and your sense of well-being.

I must emphasize that this book does not give medical advice. However, it should give you an understanding of the medical profession and serve as a realistic guide to dealing with today's health care system, so that you can work within that system from a position of knowledge and strength rather than one of ignorance, fear and weakness. In short, I hope THE DOCTOR BOOK will assist you to be at the *cause,* rather than the *effect,* of your own health care.

Wesley J. Smith
Woodland Hills, California

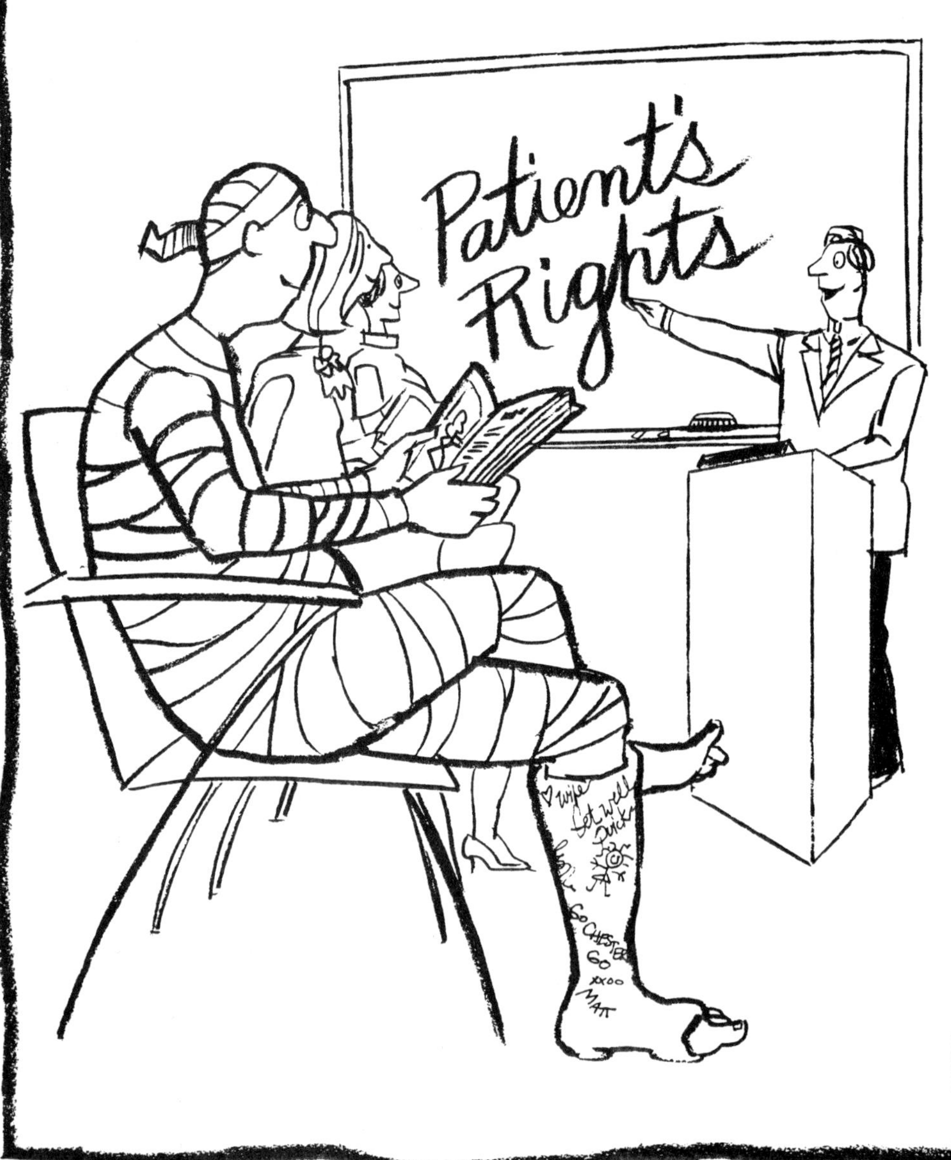
Patient's Rights
Get well
GO CHESTER GO
MATT

Introduction

It costs most families in our country a month's salary to pay for their annual health insurance and unreimbursed health products and services—and that is if everyone stays healthy.

The thrust of Wesley J. Smith's THE DOCTOR BOOK is the supremely logical belief that spending a fraction of a month's time learning about *what* you are paying for will result in better service and better health for all. This logic, however, has escaped both our educational and consumer subcultures. Young Americans spend years in school and learn little about their health, the health industry and how to use it wisely. (They learn far more about how to damage their health before, after and in between classes.) Likewise, adult consumers can attend courses on dancing, résumé writing and make-up application, but they would have to search long and far if they wanted to find classes on how to help their doctors help them or other health care related issues. As a result, patients enter this intricate medical marketplace both unknowing and vulnerable to harm and heist.

It seems unbelievable that anything as personal as being sick or injured can result in such dependency by the buyers—the very people whose bodies are the subject of all the attention—on the sellers. Lack of information regarding health, from prevention of illness to its treatment, lack of knowledge about the many pathways that patients have to negotiate with their hospitals, physicians and pharmacies, and lack of familiarity with the rights of patients to qualified, disclosed, efficient and safe care feed this passivity on the part of the consumer.

This volume, which could be called "How to Accumulate Patient Power for Your Own Well-Being in Just a Few Hours of Your Time," is your first step toward becoming an *active* player in your own health care. Smith methodically goes over your rights as a patient and your responsibilities as part of the team that works for you. He provides acute advice about how to select a physician, what constitutes a proper physical examination and what questions you need to ask your doctor in various circumstances. I think his deciphering of Medicare, Medicaid and other health insurance is particularly helpful to the millions of people who do not speak medical or legalese. You will learn that standards in hospitals and clinics exist for you to invoke and use—that you can leave the hospital knowing that you can persist in improving its operations in some way, large or small. And when things go wrong with your physician or hospital, well, Smith is a former practicing lawyer who knows what he's talking about. His section on being alert to overcharges on your medical bill provides approaches to those computerized puzzles that can alleviate your budget worries and deter future billing errors. For its wealth of this and other vital information, THE DOCTOR BOOK should be treated as a reference book and should be installed on every family's bookshelf.

Beyond that, I hope that this work by Wesley J. Smith, and those in the various reaches of medicine and health whom he consulted, stimulates you toward an even broader philosophy of health and well-being. Many important books are not particularly interesting, and when you obtain one that is both, you could be launching your mind into a readier grasp of a confident and continuing interest into the ever widening determinants of health and disease and trauma in our technological world. Over the years, I have encountered victims of accidents on the highway who became very skilled advocates of safer motor vehicle travel, from acting against drunk driving to pushing for safer automobiles. And many health advocacy groups in diverse areas of illness have been started by people who experienced these diseases or lost close relatives to them. Homemakers in communities all over the country are sounding the alert against toxic, seeping dumps, polluted air, contaminated water and radioactive power plants. They do not want to tolerate conditions that will mean more stays in hospitals, more visits to doctors and more funerals. And so the arc of health preservation becomes wider as we learn more about what distant and proximate causes lead to the major and minor diseases and casualties which the health care industry charged Americans 500 billion dollars for in 1987.

In sum, author Smith, with his easy style and humorous asides, is offering both a telescope and a microscope to bring the very blurred landscape of the business of medicine into closer and closer focus. To absorb what is written in this volume is to develop one of life's most useful skills and curiosities. And because illnesses and injuries often require prompt attention, it is prudent to read THE DOCTOR BOOK *before* you need it so you can be assured of having this important information at your fingertips; the materials in these pages are meant to foresee and forestall trouble as well as to help you respond to crises and ready you to make informed decisions and inquiries. In the process you will become a first class patient!

Ralph Nader
Washington, D.C.

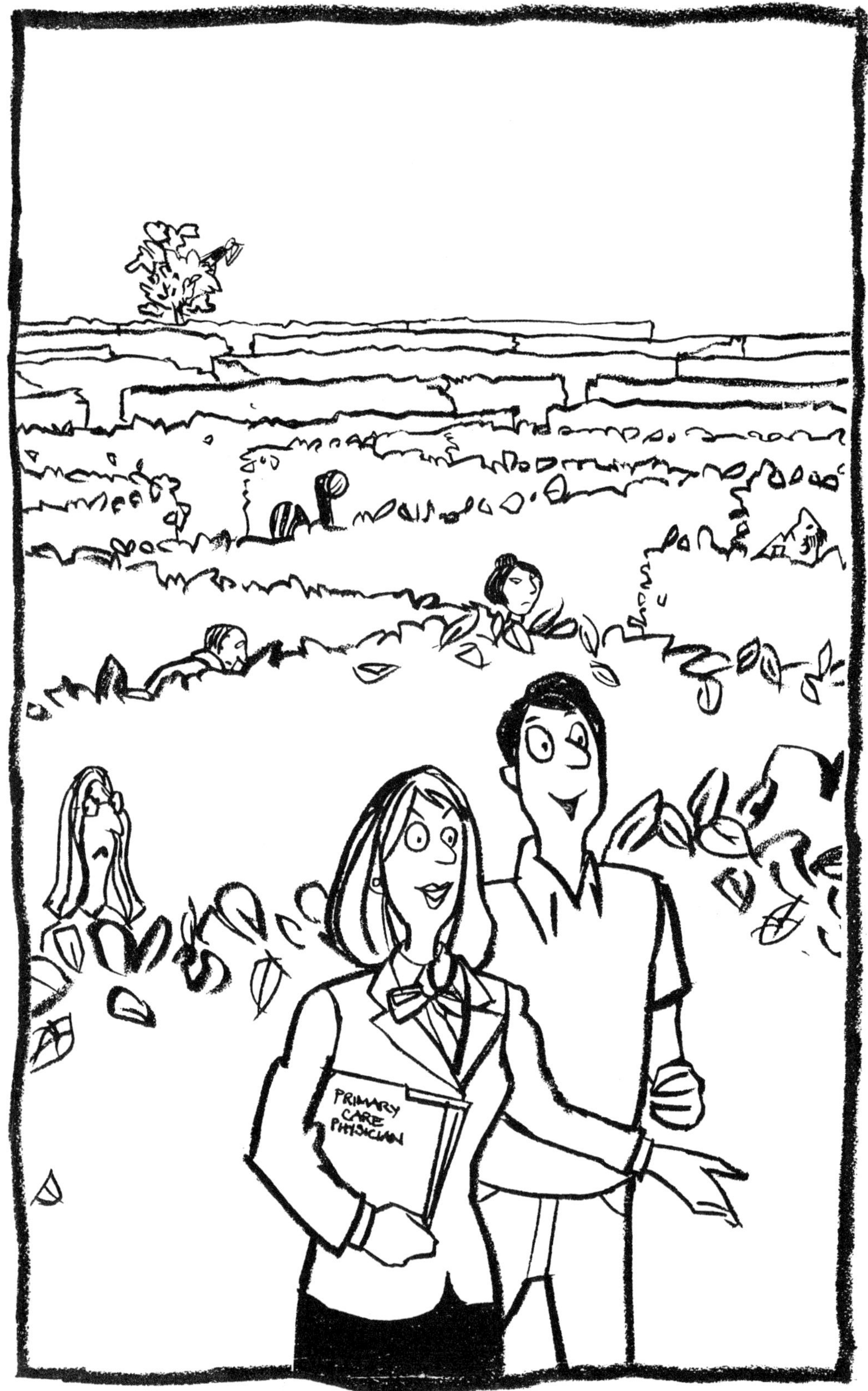
PRIMARY CARE PHYSICIAN

·1·

CHAPTER

You've Got A Friend

The Importance Of The Primary Care Physician

Now, imagine that you are suddenly transported to a mysterious land. You most certainly want a guide who will serve as an interpreter and as an advocate, someone who will act on your behalf in the event of trouble and whose sworn duty it is to help you have a safe journey.

For many of us, the "land" of health care is such a frightening and mysterious place, where "learned men and women" speak of life and death in terms we don't understand, using multisyllable words that somehow seem devoid of emotion, and so, when it comes to our own medical care, we truly need a guide to steer us through this potentially life-threatening confusion. Each of us needs an educator and advocate whose job it is to help us stay healthy and, when we are not, whose responsibility it is to assist us in receiving the best that the health care system has to offer.

Fortunately, we don't have to look very far for such a guide or advocate, for that is the duty of the primary care physician, who lives and works right in your very own community.

Introducing The PCP

All right, you ask, just who *am* I talking about? Hasn't the day of the good old general practitioner who took care of us from birth until death gone the way of the horse and carriage? Isn't medicine now in the hands of the high-powered specialist who collects diplomas the way some people collect stamps and whose humanity and compassion has been eclipsed by greed and the demands of high technology?

Well, yes and no. Yes, the day of the G.P. is indeed vanishing. But, a new breed of doctor has evolved to take his or her place. And yes, that doctor is indeed a "specialist," but not one who can't see the forest for the trees. Rather, he or she is a skilled professional whose training is specifically geared to providing you with all of the things that the old G.P. could, and more, while keeping the humanity and sense of caring that made the doctors of yesteryear seem so special. In short, the primary care physician is one who makes a "specialty" of general care.

• Just What Do They Do? •

A common misconception about primary care physicians is that they are only there to diagnose and treat illness, as in, "You've got a cold. Take two aspirin and call me in the morning." Those are indeed important functions, but in reality diagnosis and treatment are only the tip of the PCP iceberg, for your doctor's real job is to take care of the *whole* of you, not just your various parts.

Maintenance

Imagine your body as a well-tooled factory; the machinery is well-placed and hums with activity, the sales department keeps the orders coming in and the work force's morale is high. A big part of your primary care physician's job is to make sure that your "factory" stays that way. He or she accomplishes this by:

Inspection: By undergoing periodic physicals, your doctor is able to monitor the "plant" to see if any rust may be forming around the machinery and take care of it before it has a chance to create a malfunction. Beyond that, checkups allow your PCP to get a handle on what is "normal" for you so that changes are easier to spot. For example, let's say your normal blood pressure is 110/63, and has been for several years. Then, one day it is 140/88. A physician unfamiliar with you might not take note of this, as it is in the "normal" range for the adult population. But bells and sirens might be triggered in your PCP's head, since for *you* as an individual, 140/88 is high.

Hands-On Management: A good plant manager knows that the best way to prevent trouble is to head it off at the pass. If the "boiler" has had a history of overheating, special attention will be given to the gauge to make sure it doesn't enter the red zone. If labor difficulties are brewing, efforts will be made to deal with the situation before tempers flare. That's the difference between "preventive management" and "crisis management." Likewise, your PCP wants, and in fact, needs, to know a great deal about your life. And not just about the aches and pains, but about the way you live. Do you smoke? Are you happy? Is your job getting you down? Are your parents still alive? If not, what did they die from? The answers to these and other questions all help your PCP get a better understanding of who and what you are, which helps him or her practice *preventive* medicine rather than *crisis* medicine.

Making Repairs: At some point or another, even in the best-run factory, breakdowns occur which temporarily interrupt, or at the very least, slow down, production. At such times repairs must be made in the quickest possible time so that the factory's well-being as a whole does not begin to suffer. Similarly, when we become ill, it is our PCP whom we see for diagnosis and treatment to prevent minor illnesses from becoming major diseases.

Monitoring Defects: Sooner or later in any factory, even the best equipment begins to show signs of aging and slowly begins to lose its ability to function. At such times the manufacturer is forced to nurse the machinery along to keep it working as well as it can for as long as possible. And so it is that your illness or affliction may be "chronic" and have no cure, as in the case of diabetes or high blood pressure. If so, your PCP may have to monitor the condition to make sure it is under control. If it is not, your PCP will go back to the old drawing board to see what went wrong and, if possible, fix it, the focus being on maintaining your quality of life rather than searching for a cure.

Education

We like to think the human species is the most intelligent form of life in the universe. (Now there's a frightening thought!) Yet, no matter how well-educated we may be, or how experienced in the "college of hard knocks" we think we are, it is safe to say that what we as individuals don't know far exceeds all that we do know. For example, a produce supervisor may be able to talk about tomatoes for days, but knows nothing about nuclear physics, while all that a physicist with twenty university degrees may know about tomatoes is that they are red. Meanwhile, both will be largely ignorant about matters of health and medicine, and much of what they *do* know, may be in error.

That's where primary care physicians come in. A big part of their job is to educate their patients. That education can deal with lifestyle, such as a "Dutch Uncle" lecture on smoking to a five-pack-a-day man who wonders why in the world he coughs whenever he tries to laugh. Or it may come in the form of teaching a patient about a newly diagnosed disease. Perhaps it's the ob/gyn who prints a monthly medical newsletter or the pediatrician who recommends a book on sex education to an embarrassed parent. Whatever it is, if it concerns your health, your PCP has the knowledge it takes to help. So go ahead. Ask. If your PCP doesn't have the answer, he or she will be able to direct you to someone who does.

Referrals

In the beginning, there were simply doctors, who handled just about everything from childbirth to surgery. Of course, they believed in "bleeding" people with leeches to cure colds, but we won't go into that. Then, years later, doctors evolved into two groups: G.P.s, who went through medical school and internship and then hung out a shingle, and those who continued their education within a narrow and specific field in what came to be known as residency. These doctors were called "specialists."

Then the G.P.s began to fade away. They were replaced by M.D.s who practiced general care or general surgery, but who also completed residency and thus claimed the right to be called specialists, too. That created a bit of an identity crisis for the specialists because, if the general care docs and general surgeons were now called "specialists," what were the specialists going to be called? A civil war was averted with the Treaty of Hippocrates, in which it was agreed that specialists could take further training beyond normal residency in a narrowly defined field and become "sub-specialists." And so things stand today. Are you still with me?

Now, there comes into every PCP's life a case where he or she does not possess the skills or training to diagnose or treat a patient adequately. At such times, your PCP is ethically bound to advise you to get the opinion of, or treatment from, a sub-specialist. Doctors refer to this as a "consult."

For example, assume that you have a heart rhythm problem that your doctor can't control. You will be told that you should see a cardiologist, who is an internist with a sub-specialty in treating diseases of the heart.

But which cardiologist? A big city will have dozens and you will want the best one you can find. Again, your PCP can help. Part of his or her job is to know the abilities and reputations of the sub-specialists that practice within your geographic area, or on occasion, in another part of the country, and refer you to them. Of course you have the right to refuse the recommendation or to find a sub-specialist on your own, but if you trust your PCP, his or her referral can save a lot of time and aggravation. (More on this in the next chapter.)

Communication And Follow Up

Returning to the factory metaphor, your PCP can be viewed as the plant manager whom we employ to maintain and operate our factory of health, while the sub-specialist can be looked upon as the consultant who may be brought in to attend to special problems on the assembly line, a job for which he or she has been specially trained.

When it comes to discussing what is actually wrong with the assembly line, we as the factory owners may prefer to communicate with the manager we have hired, a professional whom we know and trust, rather than the consultant with whom we may not have built a rapport as yet. Both professionals know this and no one will be offended. In fact, part of the consultant's job is to write a complete report to the plant manager telling him or her all about why the assembly line looks like the classic assembly line bit from *I Love Lucy,* and to suggest what can be done to fix it.

Hand-Holding

Sometimes what we need most in life is a "professional grandmother" who can soothe our fears, hold our hand and tell us what to do to make everything all right. A big part of your PCP's job is to "be there" when you need this caring assistance.

Perhaps you are a new mother whose child preferred to have an *eraser en brochette* for lunch instead of apple sauce. Your PCP will be there to tell you that everything will come out just fine in the end. And who can the Bar-B-Q King call when he pours too much lighter fluid on the fire and burns his hand? His friendly PCP, who will tell him how to treat the burn. And we could call on our PCP for the straight scoop on the latest celebrity diet being pitched on the "Phil Donahue Show." More seriously, if you are brought to an emergency room unconscious, the E.R. staff turns first for assistance to your PCP, whose knowledge of your medical history can save time, money and even your life. Because your PCP should be there for you in time of need, seven days a week, twenty-four hours a day, he or she won't have time for the really important stuff, like making chicken soup—so leave that to your real grandmother!

Individualized Care

As a nation, we pride ourselves on our belief in the importance of each and every person. Yet, all around us the rugged individualism that we so honor seems to be losing ground to a "collectivist spirit;" as our major institutions increasingly dance to the tune of large groups, the individual can get lost in the shuffle.

Unfortunately, this same trend also seems to be occurring in health care. Medicare, for example, is now operated in part on the basis of what are called "DRGs" (diagnosis-related groups), which pay treating institutions at *predetermined* levels for the medical treatment of Medicare recipients based on the *average* cost of persons with the same diagnosis. In other words, if a Medicare beneficiary is hospitalized, payment will not be based on the *actual* cost of that individual's treatment, but on the *average* cost to treat that specific affliction around the nation. This means that the hospital's financial incentive is to discharge the patient as soon as it is medically possible, since a discharge made earlier than the average visit increases profit, and a discharge made later than this average may create a financial loss.

Where the government insurance programs tread, the private sector is sure to follow. Many health policies now require that you obtain prior approval from committees for non-emergency hospitalizations and for many surgeries as a condition for payment of full benefits. In other words, there's a whole lot of second-guessing going on.

In this environment, PCPs are increasingly forced to act as advocates of their patients. This may take the form of appealing a hospital's decision to discharge, or perhaps fighting a medical committee to get approval for specific diagnostic tests. But whatever form it takes, part of your PCP's job is to make sure that the level of your health care is based on your individual needs and not on the demands of "the bottom line."

• Who Are They? •

Today, a primary care physician can range from an internist to a family practitioner to a pediatrician—even to an ob/gyn. Your particular tastes and needs should be your guide as you choose this all-important person, and remember that *you have a choice* in this most important and fundamental health care decision.

Internists

When most people think of PCPs, they think of internists. For our purposes, we will define an internist as a doctor who makes a specialty of internal medicine. Of course, if you don't know what "internal medicine" is, you probably still don't know what I am talking about. *Internal medicine is the diagnosis, care and treatment of diseases of the body in adults, excluding surgery.* Or to put it another way, an internist will diagnose and treat but will not "cut."

> **Hint:** Many sub-specialists are increasingly practicing as primary care physicians as well as consultants, due to the increase in competition within the health care system. If an internist whom you may wish to serve as your PCP is also a sub-specialist such as a gastroenterologist, make sure that he or she really enjoys the burdens of primary care. Otherwise, you could get short-changed.

Family Practitioners

Family practice is the newest specialty on the block, one designed to fill the vacuum left by the near extinction of the G.P. A family practitioner, unlike an internist, will conduct some general surgery and will treat children. In fact, a family practitioner's training includes pediatrics, surgery, internal medicine, obstetrics and gynecology and psychiatry.

An interesting note about family care specialists: As you will learn (if you don't already know) the different medical disciplines (i.e., internal medicine, pediatrics, surgery) "certify" a practitioner's "knowledge in each field", which is tested by what are called "the boards." When a physician passes the Family Practice boards he or she is then called "Board Certified" by the American Board of Family Practice, the only specialty board that requires recertification—every seven years—and also requires a specified amount of continuing medical education within the family practice field as a condition of that recertification. (Many states also require continuing education as a condition of a physician's license to practice, but this is not the same since the requirements are less demanding and the education need not even be in the field of the physician's specialty.)

Pediatricians

A pediatrician treats children from birth through their late teens and sometimes even into their early twenties. In essence, a pediatrician is an internist for children, although many will perform minor surgery, such as putting in stitches or draining abscesses. In addition, a large part of a pediatrician's job is to educate parents on their children's health care and to deal with behavioral issues which may have little to do with illness, but a lot to do with the child as a "whole person."

Ob/Gyns

Short for obstetrician/gynecologist, these physicians, unlike Prissy of *Gone With The Wind* fame, definitely know something about "birthin' babies" and also care for the female reproductive system. Also, while ob/gyns are not technically primary care physicians, many women prefer to use them as such.

More on family practitioners, internists, pediatricians and ob/gyns in Chapter 2.

Now, many of you may still be asking, "But which of the PCPs is best?" My answer is, "It depends." (How's that for being helpful?) What you have to ask yourself is this: What is more important to me as a patient—*depth* or *breadth*? For example, if *convenience* is a big issue in your life, you may wish to look for a primary care physician who can treat a broader range of ailments without having to refer you to a sub-specialist. This would probably be a *family care specialist.* Meanwhile, your best friend's need is for a physician with *depth* of knowledge. He or she may prefer to work with a physician who treats a narrower scope of afflictions than with a doctor who has trained in areas of medicine which do not concern him or her, such as pediatrics. Thus, his or her choice for a PCP would probably be an *internist.* Parents may prefer that their children be treated by a doctor who only treats children—a *pediatrician*—or they may feel it is important that each family member have the same doctor—a *family care specialist.* And, as I said earlier, some women may have such a strong rapport with their gynecologists that they prefer to keep all of their health care in the hands of this one physician, and thus will also utilize their *ob/gyn* for primary care. So, you see, it all depends on your particular needs.

NOTES TO THE CHART*

The primary care physician can truly be your savior. My most important function as a primary care physician is, in my opinion, when a sudden illness or an emergency strikes one of my patients.

Medical emergencies are always frightening, even for us physicians. But there is a difference in how doctors and laypersons respond to the problem. Because of my training and experience, I can usually differentiate between truly life-threatening problems and medical matters that need attention, but which are not likely to result in permanent harm. Laypersons don't have this vantage point so are more likely to overreact to relatively minor concerns.

A telephone call to your physician will immediately give you the same edge I already have by putting you in touch with an expert who will know what to do in the circumstances you are presented with. A matter that needs attention, but which is not a true emergency, can probably be handled immediately by your own doctor, who will try to squeeze you in. This gives you the advantage of being treated by someone who knows you as an individual and not just as a name on a chart.

Likewise, in a true emergency, you will be directed to call the paramedics, and your doctor will coordinate your care with the emergency room personnel, informing them about your (or your family member's) health history and your unique medical circumstances. This not only saves time, but could save your life by allowing the emergency team to get right to the probable cause of your distress, rather than by wasting time in what may be a lengthy diagnostic process.

*NOTES TO THE CHART *are the comments of Dr. Daniel V. Ehrensaft, M.D., a board certified physician in the fields of internal medicine and infectious diseases who practices in Los Angeles.*

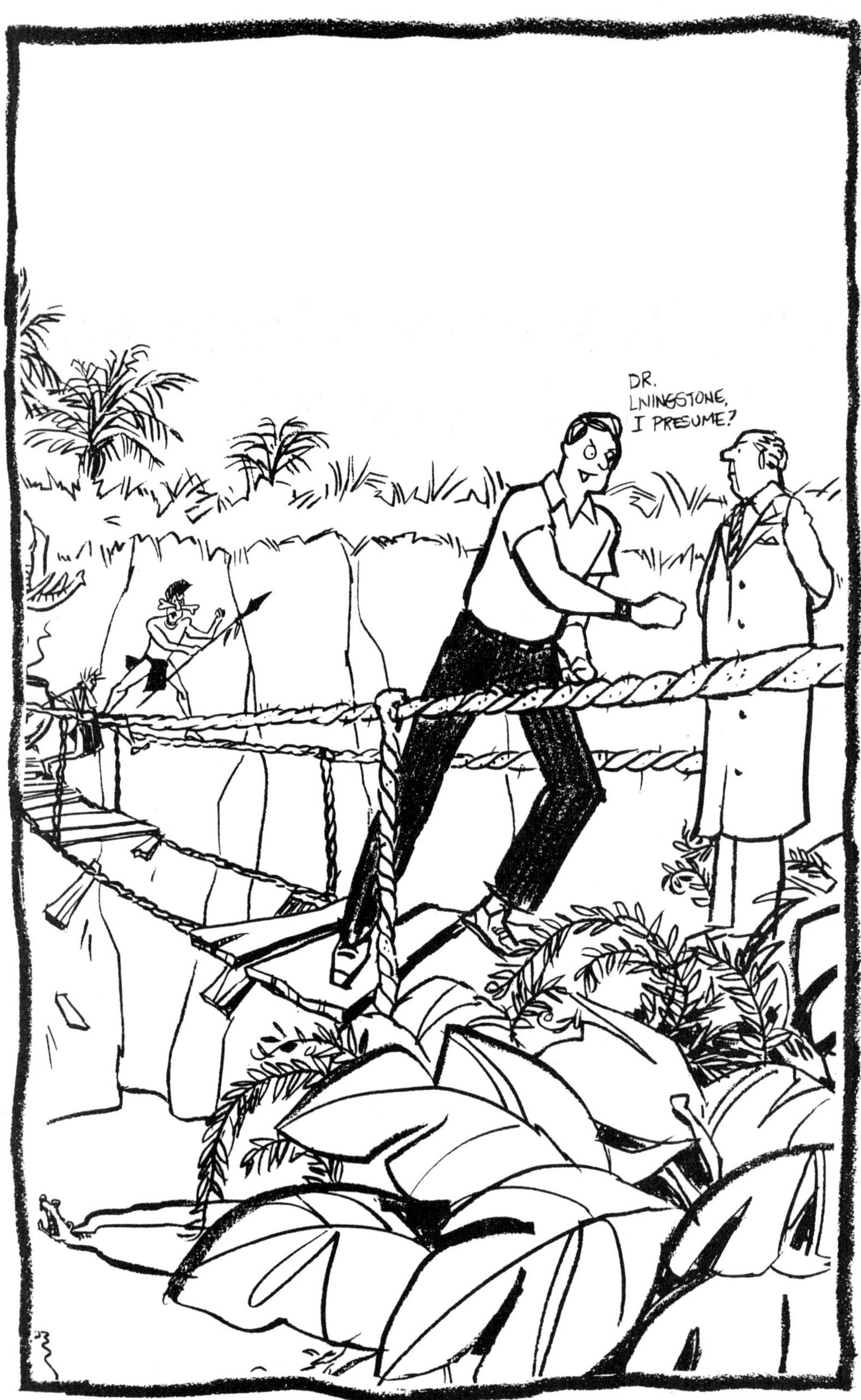
DR. LIVINGSTONE, I PRESUME?

·2·

CHAPTER

Climb Every Mountain, Ford Every Stream

Finding The Right Doctor

Each of us has different attitudes and opinions about the *kind of person* our doctor should be. You might believe, for example, that a doctor should possess the personal warmth and courage of a Captain James T. Kirk of *Star Trek* fame, while I might prefer the cool scientific approach of a Mr. Spock, and someone else's ideal physician would be a doctor with an intense passion for healing, like Leonard "Bones" McCoy. Thus the doctor who may be right for you may not be right for me, and neither of our choices would suit your friend down the block.

Show business characters aside, what are the qualities to look for in a prospective doctor? One of the doctors I spoke with said that a doctor should be a "loving healer." Another expert advised that the doctor should be a good diagnostician. Perhaps the best way I heard it put was "Find a doctor who meets the "5 A*s*." A doctor who meets these "5 A*s*" is one who is:

- Able
- Available
- Accessible
- Affable
- Affordable

Ability is the threshold question each patient should be concerned with before everything else, and concerns the doctor's professional or clinical skills. For example, does the doctor have sufficient *credentials* in the field of care you need to be trusted with your health? Has the doctor kept up on the latest diagnostic tests and techniques? In short, does he or she possess good "doctoring skills?" If not, that doctor is not for you.

Availability: A doctor can be the best in the world but will do you no good if he or she is not reasonably available to treat or consult with you. Thus, if a doctor keeps severely restricted office hours or is not available after hours for urgent concerns, you may wish to continue looking.

Accessibility means that the doctor practices in a place you can get to. If you are dependent on the bus to get to the doctor's office, for example, you probably won't want to choose a doctor two miles from the nearest bus stop or one which takes forever to reach. Or, if you are on a tight budget and your doctor does not validate for parking, perhaps the fifteen or twenty dollars it would cost to park would keep you from going at all. I could think of many other examples, but the principle would be the same in each case. With rare exceptions, such as when you need a sub-sub-sub-specialist, you are better off choosing a doctor whom you can see with relative comfort and ease.

Affordability does not need much explanation—a doctor should work within your financial means. Thus, if you are on Medicare, you may want a doctor who will accept what Medicare sets as a reasonable fee. If you are on a tight budget, you will need a doctor who will permit you to make monthly payments. What good does it do you to have a doctor you can't use because you can't afford the bill?

Affability means a lot more than just being a nice person. It means effective communication skills, it means treating a patient with respect, it means caring about the patient's outcome. In short, affability is a word which is sometimes expressed in the phrase "bedside manner" or "the art of medicine," each of which is required if a physician is to really earn our trust.

•Taking One Step At A Time•

The question, then, is how do we go about finding a doctor who corresponds with our own personal tastes? Well, there isn't a single "right" method to choosing a doctor any more than there is a single way to decorate a home or cook a steak. There are, however, certain ways to go about the task that are definitely better than others, so let's get to it. (By the way, those of you of the "open a phone book, close your eyes and point" persuasion can skip to the next chapter, since we won't be discussing your technique.)

Step 1: Choose The Right Kind of Doctor

An ancient Chinese proverb says that the longest journey begins with the first step. When it comes to selecting a doctor, that first step is identifying the *kind* of doctor you want. This isn't an easy task considering the difficulty (and danger) of self-diagnosis, although it is safe to say that someone suffering from the symptoms of hemorrhoids is not going to need an "ear, nose and throat" specialist.

Before we start, let's define some of the terminology we will be using. Basically, doctors in each field come in three different forms: Residents—doctors who have passed medical school and internship, and who are now undergoing clinical training in the specific discipline in which they intend to practice; Board Qualified Physicians—doctors who have completed their residency (which generally takes three to five years, depending on the field) but who have not taken or passed their "boards" or perhaps have even flunked the boards; and Board Certified Physicians—doctors who have completed their residency and passed their boards, which usually consist of a written and oral exam in the specific field in which the doctor wishes to practice.

> **Hint:** Doctors can legally call themselves "specialists" in a given area even if they have no credentials in the field. Thus, when asking whether a doctor is qualified by training to treat you, don't ask, "Are you a specialist?" Instead ask, "*Are you board certified*?" If you find that the physician is not at least board qualified, he or she may not be a qualified specialist after all.

The following is a general summary of the various medical fields that exist in the United States. You will note that some areas overlap with others, which isn't surprising considering that medicine is at best an inexact science.

Family Practice: A family practitioner is a physician who specializes in general family care. A family practice specialist will have training in internal medicine, general surgery, obstetrics and gynecology, pediatrics and psychiatry.

Internal Medicine: An internist is a physician who diagnoses and "medically" (i.e., non-surgically) treats diseases of adults. Internists frequently work as primary care physicians.

Many internists also take advanced residencies in specific areas. Upon completion, they become board qualified or, if they pass further tests, board certified *sub-specialists.* And so they become experts in a narrow field and will know that field "inside and out." (Pardon the pun.) These sub-specialties are:

Cardiology–the treatment of the heart and vascular system (blood vessels).

Endocrinology–the treatment of metabolic diseases such as diabetes and diseases of the thyroid and other glands.

Gastroenterology–the treatment of diseases of the digestive system, most frequently of the stomach, liver and intestines.

Hematology–the treatment of afflictions and diseases of the blood.

Infectious Disease–the treatment of diseases and afflictions caused by microorganisms such as viruses or bacteria, whether or not they are "communicable."

Oncology–cancer treatment, such as through the use of chemotherapy.

Nephrology–the treatment of diseases of the kidneys.

Pulmonary Disease–the treatment of diseases of the lungs.

Rheumatology–the treatment of arthritis.

General Surgery: Physicians with a specialty in surgery perform general abdominal operations, lumpectomies, breast surgery and a wide variety of other procedures.

There are also several surgical sub-specialties. Many of these cover the same "body parts" as the internal medicine sub-specialties because some diseases must be treated surgically rather than through medication. (By the way, a board qualified surgical sub-specialist who is also board certified in general surgery, will have spent up to *eight* years in surgical residency! No wonder they charge so much!)

Head and Neck Surgery–formerly called ear, nose and throat surgery, this surgical sub-specialty deals with surgical procedures of the head and neck such as a thyroidectomy.

Neurosurgery–surgery involving the brain, such as the removal of a tumor.

Orthopedics–operations on bones or joints, such as a hip replacement.

Plastic Surgery–also known as reconstructive surgery, plastic surgery involves the repair of injured or deformed body parts, as well as the more commonly known cosmetic procedures like "chin tucks," "face peels" and rhinoplasty, or as it is called commonly, a nose job.

Hint: There are physicians who perform cosmetic plastic surgery who are not qualified by experience or training to do so. Before you agree to any such procedure, make sure your physician has the appropriate qualifications to perform the surgery. The face you save may be your own.

Thoracic Surgery–surgery of the lungs and heart, such as replacing a defective heart valve.

Vascular Surgery–surgery of the blood vessels, such as a heart bypass operation or a procedure to remove varicose veins.

Obstetrics/Gynecology: These physicians care for and treat the female reproductive system by surgery, i.e., removing cysts or tumors, through preventive tests such as Pap smears, and through the prescribing of medications, such as hormones or birth control pills. Obstetricians also care for pregnant women and deliver babies.

Pediatrics: Pediatricians care for and treat children from birth through the teens or early twenties. There are also pediatric sub-specialties, for example pediatric surgery, and even what might be called sub-sub-specialties such as pediatric orthopedic surgery.

Urology: Considered by many to be the male equivalent of the ob/gyn, urologists actually do much more, treating diseases of the urinary tract in both men and women as well as providing prostate care for men. Urologists treat both medically and surgically.

Neurology: The medical treatment of diseases of the nervous system, such as epilepsy and Parkinson's disease. Neurologists do not perform surgery.

Dermatology: Surgical and medical treatment of afflictions and diseases of the skin, such as cancer or acne.

Psychiatry: Not to be confused with psychologists, who do not attend medical school, psychiatrists are M.D.s who treat behavioral disorders of the mind, such as depression or schizophrenia.

Anesthesiology: When you "haven't got time for the pain," the anesthesiologist is the physician who administers the drugs that keep it at bay, usually during an operation. A less well-known function of these highly trained specialists is their responsibility for the very life of the patient during surgery, which ranges from monitoring vital signs to deciding whether to terminate the procedure if the patient is in distress.

Emergency Medicine: At one time, many emergency rooms were attended by physicians from different disciplines who were moonlighting to earn a little extra money to pay bills. No more. Today emergency medicine is a board certified specialty with residency requirements and test procedures all its own. As you might expect, E.R. physicians are trained in a wide variety of disciplines—from trauma care to cardiology—which makes your trip to the emergency room much safer than it used to be.

Physical Medicine: This field of medical care, which includes physical therapy and "sports medicine," has been growing as those of us over thirty continue to hurt ourselves by trying to act as if we were twenty. On a more serious note, physicians who practice physical medicine also care for the seriously injured and the bodily impaired.

Pathology: Patients rarely interact with pathologists, at least not when they are capable of exchanging a handshake, since these doctors are responsible for performing autopsies. Pathologists also test tissues from living patients, such as checking the results of a biopsy to determine whether a growth is cancerous.

Even though I haven't listed every type of medical field there is (no slight intended), you can see that medicine truly is a very specialized profession. That can be very frightening to people who don't know what kind of doctor to select and who don't have a PCP to treat them or point them in the right direction. Is there anything they can do besides panic? You betcha, and here's my prescription:

• If you are feeling very ill or fear that something is seriously wrong, "get thee to an emergency room" as soon as possible. There you will be examined and referred to the specialist "on call" if that should prove to be necessary. More about that later.

• There are also "urgent care," or ambulatory care centers popping up all over the place which accept walk-ins. If you feel ill, but don't feel like it's a real emergency, try one of them.

• If you are not ill, but feel that something just isn't right, a family care specialist or an internist is probably a good place to start. If he or she can't find the problem, they will then be more than happy to refer you to the appropriate physician, and, in the meantime, you may have found your PCP.

Step 2: Get Referrals

When it comes to selecting a doctor, you definitely do not have to rely on luck, nor do you have to count on your fingers to "do the walking through the Yellow Pages." That's because there is an abundance of good solid sources of referrals who can direct you to good qualified physicians. All you have to be willing to do is take the time to look.

Other Doctors: The first and probably best place to turn when looking for the name of a good doctor is another doctor. Most physicians are aware of the reputations of other doctors within the local medical community and thus know which physicians should be recommended and which avoided. *This should be especially true of your PCP* (if you have one) whose job it is to refer you to the best sub-specialists available when your problem needs the input of an outside expert.

Hint: Many of the physicians I spoke with complained that some doctors don't make referrals based on medical excellence but rather, on social contacts or as part of a "mutual referral society." In fact, more than one doctor noted with some irony that there are some physicians who refer family members to them but not patients. Thus, when a recommendation is made, ask the following questions:

Why have you recommended this particular physician over all of the others in town?

What are his or her credentials?

Are there others whom I can talk to about this particular physician's reputation and skills?

Have you ever referred members of your own family to this doctor?

It might also be a good idea to get the names of three physicians so that you can compare and contrast their credentials and personal attributes for yourself.

Nurses and Other Medical Personnel: It often seems that nurses, medical secretaries, office managers and others who serve as support staff in the world of medicine are seen far more often than they are heard. That is not to say, however, that they don't hear what is going on around them. On the contrary, ask any office manager which doctors he or she would recommend or avoid in the local medical community, and you are sure to get an earful! And, if you are fortunate enough to know someone who works in the health field, don't hesitate to ask for a referral or about a particular physician's reputation. You might also ask these contacts to ask their boss for his or her opinion. After all, it's better to be safe than sorry.

Friends and Family Members: I am a strong believer that other consumers are a very reliable source of information about products and services. If you are going to buy a new car, for example, and you have a friend who owns a model that you are thinking of selecting, you will naturally ask that friend for his or her opinion about that particular vehicle. If your friend tells you that the car stalls in the mornings and is always in the shop, chances are you will scratch that model off your list of potential candidates. On the other hand, if your friend is going to nominate the car for the "Automotive Hall Of Fame," you will probably make a beeline to the nearest showroom.

This is equally true in the field of medicine. In fact, referrals from satisfied patients are a principal way doctors build a successful medical practice. (Don't forget, doctors in private practice may be "professionals" but they are also entrepreneurs.) So, conduct your own market survey. If you are looking for a PCP, ask your friends and relatives if they would recommend theirs. If your cousin had a surgery similar to the one you may be facing, ask if she liked her surgeon. And always remember to say the magic word, "*Why*?" Compare models and prices, and then make your selection. I'll bet you won't end up with a lemon.

Local Medical Societies: If you have just moved to a new community and don't know anybody, or even if you have been a lifelong resident, there is a place in town you can turn to for referrals, and that is your local county medical association. These voluntary organizations are made up of physicians who live and practice locally, and while their principal purpose is to serve the professional needs of their members, most county medical associations have computerized referral services available free or at nominal cost. The referral will normally consist of three doctors who practice in the specialty that you want close to where you live, and it will tell you where each doctor attended medical school and whether that physician is board certified in his or her specialty.

Hint: In today's climate of fear about AIDS, not all physicians will treat those unfortunate souls who have been stricken by this disease. As a result, some county associations have now added a new category to their referral lists—"will treat AIDS." So if you or someone you know has AIDS or has been exposed to the disease and has been unable to find medical help, it will probably be available through your local county medical association.

Hospitals: As competition increases in the medical profession, many hospitals now offer doctor referral services. This helps you because you have easy access to doctors who have undergone some screening for quality (sometimes more, sometimes less), and it helps the hospital because the doctors on the referral list will have "staff privileges" (i.e., they can admit and treat patients in that hospital), so if you are ever hospitalized, guess in which one it will be.

University Medical Schools: If you live close to a large university medical school and still have been unable to find a doctor with whom you are happy, try calling the head of the clinical residency program and ask if he or she can recommend someone who practices near you who possesses exceptional clinical skills.

Local Referral Services: Many areas have local referral services, usually affiliated with local hospitals, which can refer you to physicians on staff at the hospitals who sponsor the program. This service is generally provided free to the consumer. The level of pre-screening will vary.

Hint: Don't make the mistake of utilizing these referral sources as if they each exist in a vacuum. In other words, use more than one source so that you can find the names of several qualified doctors who practice in your area in order that you might have a choice. Thus, if your friend recommends a certain sub-specialist to you, run that name by your PCP. If a sub-specialist you know has recommended a primary care physician, ask your friends if they have ever heard of that doctor. By taking your time in selecting your doctor and by using all of the referral sources at your disposal, you increase the odds of finding the physician who will be just right for you.

Step 3: Research The Candidates

There is a lot of information you should have about the physicians you are thinking of selecting before you set up appointments to meet them. Happily, most of the work can be done by phone.

1. Telephone your state medical licensing board and ask whether the doctor you are interested in has ever been disciplined by the state for unprofessional conduct. As you will see in Chapter 11, it takes a lot for a physician to be subjected to professional discipline, but when it does happen, it becomes a matter of public record (which you are entitled to find out about). Many states will also tell you whether an official investigation is pending against a particular physician, and since such matters frequently take years to reach completion, it's always a good idea to ask about "open files" as well as whether discipline has actually been imposed.

2. Contact your county medical association and ask whether the physicians on your list are members in good standing. Of course, the mere fact of membership alone is no guarantee that the doctor is a good one or that you will have a positive experience, but it may indicate that the doctor has a sense of idealism and commitment to the profession since membership costs money in the form of dues and time in the form of committee assignments and membership meetings. (Of course, some doctors join for the sheer purpose of drumming up business.)

Regardless of the reasons for joining, membership also implies that the doctor is sensitive to peer review since local medical associations usually investigate and act upon ethical complaints, such as fee disputes or poor service, which are not serious enough to cost a doctor his or her license to practice (see Chapter 11).

Most local associations should also be able to supply the physician's credentials (i.e., whether the doctor is board certified) and office hours, whether foreign languages are spoken in his or her office and whether he or she is willing to take Medicare or Medicaid patients.

Hint: When you contact the medical association, ask whether a member physician is on the referral list. If not, it may mean nothing, since not all doctors wish to receive referrals—but it could mean that the association has serious ethical questions about the doctor in question and has removed him or her from the referral list. Thus, if you find that a member doctor you are investigating is not on the referral list, ask the association, "Why not?"

---

3. Call the physician's office and ask the staff personnel what the office hours are, whether parking is provided or validated (validations can save you a lot of money over the years) and whether there are facilities for the handicapped in the building, if that is important to you. The staff will also usually be able to tell you what the doctor's credentials are, whether the doctor assists in the preparation of insurance forms and whether there is a charge for the service and whether the doctor will accept patients on Medicare or Medicaid. *You can also find out if the doctor accepts assignment of health insurance benefits or expects you to pay in advance*, an important consideration for patients on a limited budget.

4. Go to your local library and look up in one or both of the following books the doctors you are thinking about retaining: *The American*

Medical Association Directory of Physicians, which lists every doctor in the country, or the *Directory of Medical Specialists,* which lists every doctor with a board certification, along with credentials. If the doctor is not listed in one of these books, either he or she is relatively new to the practice of medicine or something is wrong.

Step 4: Interview The Physicians On Your List

No matter how diligent you are in searching for the names of the best physicians in town and no matter how deeply you research each candidate, you cannot possibly make an informed and intelligent decision as to which doctor to choose until you've had a chance to get a feel for the "human being" underneath the white coat and stethoscope. (Yes, doctors *are* human.) The only way to do that is to meet them face-to-face. This means, of course, you will have to schedule an appointment.

Hint: Sometimes you can get a feel for a person over the telephone, so before you meet the doctor, try to arrange a phone conference first. If the doctor is unfriendly, rude or won't talk to you at all, it is probably a good idea to scratch him or her off your list. I mean, if they treat you that way before you "sign along for the cruise," imagine how they will treat you once you've been hooked and landed.

It's always a good idea to ask ahead of time what you will need to bring with you. This will usually include some or all of the following:

- Proof of insurance
- Past medical records, depending on the situation
- A list of the medications you are taking, along with their dosage and the number of times you take the medicine per day—or easier still, bring your medicine along with you
- A complete list of allergies, if any

Hint: If you have been referred by your primary care physician or other treating professional, be sure that doctor has communicated with the new doctor about your case and forwarded your records ahead of time. You might even volunteer your services as courier to make sure the job gets done.

It's also a good idea to write down everything you want to talk with the doctor about ahead of time, along with a list of questions you want to ask, just so you don't forget.

You should also be prepared to talk about your family's medical history, since an understanding of the past is frequently an indispensable diagnostic tool in determining what the problem is at present or what it may be in the future.

One other important point: I firmly believe you need to talk to several doctors before you choose the right one for you. Remember, medical expertise is only part of the game. You also want a doctor whom you can trust with your most intimate secrets and who will communicate openly and clearly with you about your own health. If you "look before you leap," your chances of finding Dr. Right are greatly improved. This is especially true when you are selecting a primary care physician since that relationship will be long-term and is of such fundamental importance.

Hint: Many doctors will not give free initial office consultations while others will, so be sure to ask the office policy ahead of time. If a doctor won't see you for free, ask for an appointment for a "short consultation" time. The cost will be around $40 or $50 for twenty or thirty minutes of the doctor's time, but I think it's definitely worth the price. After all, the cost of selecting the *wrong* doctor can be much, much higher.

Once you meet the doctor, you should be prepared to discuss your case in a clear and intelligent manner. The easiest way to do this is to *write down everything you want to tell or ask the doctor ahead of time* so you don't forget. It's also a good idea to take notes about what your doctor tells you—again, so you don't forget.

• Let's Play "Ten" Questions •

The following is a list of ten questions that you will probably want to ask your doctor. Of course, the list is not nor can it be all-inclusive, so don't hesitate to ask questions of your own.

1. What are your credentials?

Of all the "5 A*s*" listed at the start of this chapter, *ability* has to be the most important. After all, a pleasing and caring personality is terrific, but it won't do you much good if the doctor can't make a correct diagnosis. Besides, the very purpose of credentials is to give you, the patient, an objective way to judge whether your doctor's got "the right stuff." Here are some things to look for:

Medical School: If your doctor attended a major American or Canadian university medical school, then at least you know that he or she had the scholastic ability we all want our doctors to possess. That, of course, does not guarantee that the doctor is good. And I am not saying that doctors trained overseas or in one of the Caribbean medical schools will not be good doctors either, but I do think it is safe to say that the intellectual requirements of those schools vary greatly from institution to institution.

Residency: If your doctor successfully completed a residency at a major teaching hospital, it tells you that at the very least he or she possessed a level of clinical ability sufficient to finish training in a specialty.

Board Certification: As we've discussed, a board certified specialist or sub-specialist has completed a residency and passed examinations designed to test his or her knowledge of that specialty. If your doctor is not board certified, ask why not. It could be that he or she has chosen not to take the test, or perhaps did take it and failed. In any event, you will want your doctor to be at least board qualified in that specialty, since it is the only way you can tell whether the doctor has received sufficient training in the field.

Hint: Some specialties now offer their practitioners recertification programs. If your doctor has been recertified, it will indicate that he or she has kept on top of the field and passed another test. And it will also tell you something about the depth of his or her commitment to medicine, since with the exception of family practice, the programs are strictly voluntary.

Fellowship: Some physicians receive recognition from their peers, usually for research or other intellectual endeavors called a "fellowship." You can tell if your doctor's a fellow by looking at his or her business card. For example, a surgeon's card might read, "M.D., F.A.C.S.," for Medical Doctor, Fellow of the American College of Surgeons. (And you thought all of those initials were just for show.)

2. In which hospitals do you have staff privileges?

Many people think that every doctor can practice in every hospital. On the contrary, doctors must apply for "staff privileges," after which there is a screening process conducted by medical committees who demand a certain level of medical excellence, which are admittedly higher in some institutions than in others. (One positive aspect of the "malpractice crisis" is that it is forcing hospitals to demand higher standards of excellence in physicians who are granted staff privileges.) Thus, if your doctor is on staff in all of the major hospitals in your area, it tells you something. On the other hand, if the only hospital in which a prospective physician can practice is a forty-bed facility that he or she partially owns, that tells you something too.

Hint: If you really want to be aggressive, ask if the doctor has ever been thrown off the staff of a hospital. A "yes" should cause you to dig deeper, since it is easier to get on staff than it is to be thrown off, meaning there may have been a very good reason which you will want to know.

3. What kind of continuing education activities do you pursue?

Medicine is always in the process of explosive change, and thus a big part of your doctor's job is to keep up to date on all of the developments in his or her area of expertise. This task is accomplished by attending seminars, taking classes, "networking" and reading "the literature." If you find that the doctor doesn't take that aspect of the job seriously or if you find that your doctor resents this question or is vague in answering, you may want to think twice before "signing on the dotted line." After all, who wants a doctor who is behind the times?

4. What is my care going to cost?

Doctors in private practice wear two hats: that of the learned professional and that of the entrepreneur. That means you are going to have to pay for the services your doctor provides, partially if you have health insurance, completely if you don't. You certainly have the right to be informed ahead of time how much your care or treatment is going to cost so that you can be prepared to pay the bill.

Hint: Most doctors know they charge more than the general public can afford to pay in one lump sum and thus many will accept monthly payments or credit cards to help ease the pain. However, not all do, so if this is an important issue in your decision-making process, be sure to find out each doctor's policy ahead of time.

5. What is included in my plan of care?

Whether you are dealing with a PCP or a surgeon, you get only so much "bang" for your buck. Thus, if you are needing surgery, ask the surgeon what is included in the price, i.e., follow-up visits, telephone calls, etc. If you are retaining a primary care physician, make sure that doctor is willing to provide all of the services you expect of a PCP (see

Chapter 1). In other words, you have the right to know what services are included and what services are à la carte.

Hint: Doctors, unlike lawyers, usually don't charge for routine phone calls. However, there are those who do, so be sure to find out the office policy ahead of time to avoid an unpleasant surprise down the line.

---

6. What is your policy regarding the time for telephone calls?

Practicing medicine is not a nine-to-five occupation and most doctors know it. However, many doctors do try to organize their day so that they can handle non-emergency calls in an organized fashion. Thus, one of the things you should be sure to find out beforehand is the doctor's specific office policy regarding phone calls so that you will know how to reach your doctor in time of need.

Hint: Hand-holding is one of the bigger jobs that pediatricians perform for parents; thus many will have specific hours during the day which are set aside exclusively for phone calls. If yours does, try hard to honor that policy and limit your "information please" calls to the specified time (emergencies excepted). Not only will it make your pediatrician's job easier, but also the staff 's.

Hint: Most doctors have "beepers" so they can be reached any time of the day or night. Thus, you should not only make a point of having your doctor's phone number immediately available to you, but you should know the beeper number as well. In an emergency, the time saved could be important.

---

7. Who covers for you?

While it is true that a doctor is never off-duty, it is also true that a doctor cannot always be available in time of need. Thus, most doctors work out agreements with other doctors to cover for them during those times they are unavailable (such as when they attend that important seminar on "communicable diseases of the big toe" in Bermuda).

The key question to ask your doctor about a substitute physician is whether the substitute has the same skills that your own doctor has. After all, if you have selected a board certified gastroenterologist to help you with your digestive problems, you deserve better than relying on a second-year resident in internal medicine to treat you if your physician is sick or out of town.

8. Are you available in emergencies?
This question is important, especially in the selection of a primary care physician. Remember, an emergency can strike any time of the day or night. If it does, you will want to be able to reach your doctor immediately so that he or she can tell you what to do, whether to call the paramedics or go to an emergency room, or even just to calm you down with the reassuring news that you have overreacted to a medical problem that is not an emergency at all. Also, you will want assurances that in the event of urgent need (non-life-threatening) your doctor will be able to see you immediately, either by squeezing you in or rearranging patients with less pressing concerns. (Which also implies that you will be understanding if you are the patient whose appointment gets rearranged.)

9. What is your philosophy about ____?
Each of us has our own individual approach to health care. So do doctors. Thus, if you want a doctor who downplays medication and stresses nutrition, you should discuss that issue ahead of time. Likewise, if you are an expectant mother and believe that breast-feeding your infant is important, you will want a pediatrician or family care specialist who will work with you in implementing your desires. Obviously, the time to find out if you and your doctor are on the same wavelength is *before* you "tie the knot" and not after. Thus, if you have strong feelings about an aspect of your health care, be sure to lay it on the table so you are not disappointed down the line.

10. Do you like being a doctor?
The profession of being a doctor is thought of as one of dedication and high purpose, not to mention high money. But there can also be a downside—stress, overwork, family problems caused by frequent absence, the burden of the responsibility for the lives and well-being of others—any or all of these can eventually extract a price, which carries the generic name "burnout," from the physician.

Burnout can express itself in many ways, none of which are good news for patients. It can take the form of alcoholism, substance abuse or depression. Sometimes the victim of burnout will have a difficult time paying attention to details, or harbor a general feeling of hostility toward patients. Whatever form it takes, the existence of burnout will reduce your doctor's effectiveness in caring for you and your health.

Thus, when you ask this question, pay attention to what is being said between the lines. If you get the distinct feeling that the physician *is* unhappy in his or her work or would rather be sailing the Pacific than treating you, you might want to look elsewhere, because when a doctor suffers burnout, it is often the patient who feels the pain.

Finally, you will of course want to discuss any immediate medical problems you are having with the doctor. However, for the purposes of organization, we'll deal with those issues in future chapters as they become relevant.

• It's Decision Time, Folks •

By this time you should have a pretty good idea about the type of doctor you want and which of the candidates you interviewed has made the best impression on you, both as a healer and as a human being. So as you make your decision, balance the good points of each against the not-so-good points and "go for it," because now the real fun begins.

NOTES TO THE CHART

It has been my experience that patients frequently choose doctors for the wrong reasons. Sometimes it's because the doctor goes to the same church or synagogue, or is a member of the same fraternal order or service club. At other times a patient may decide to select a doctor because of a slick advertisement or because the doctor looked good on television.

The rationale behind these decisions, in my opinion, concerns the patient's deep desire to find a doctor that he or she can *trust.* Unfortunately, the criterion utilized to find a trustworthy physician is often insufficient to assure quality of care and only serves to lead the patient down a garden path.

The fact of the matter is, there are no shortcuts or magic formulas when it comes to selecting a good doctor. It requires the time and effort outlined in this chapter to really do the job right. So don't settle for "potluck," but be thorough in your search. Your reward will be the protection of your most valuable asset—your health.

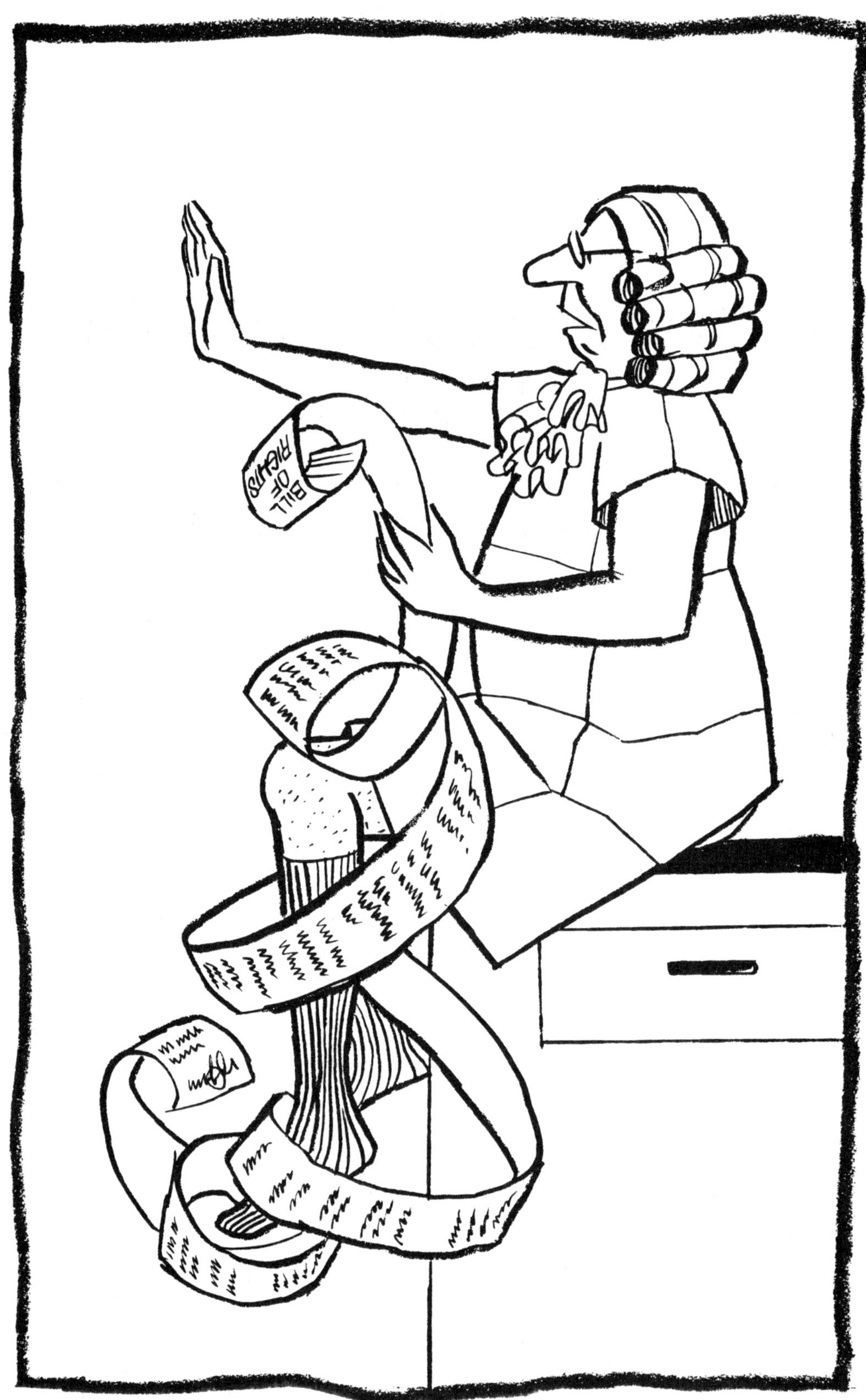
BILL
OF
RIGHTS

·3·

CHAPTER

The Patient's Bill Of Rights

Conduct You Deserve From Your Doctor

A major message of the consumer movement that has been sweeping the country in recent years is that each of us can benefit from *being at the cause* of the events of our lives rather than only *at the effect.* This idea is especially important in the field of medicine, where so much is at stake and where too many of us feel we have no rights, no power and no say in what will be done to our bodies. Happily, as you will see, we *do.*

Let's call this concept "patient power." Its purpose is to ensure that you as a patient obtain medical care that is of the highest quality and that preserves your sense of self and your dignity as a human being.

Some of the concepts we will be discussing are already embodied in law. Others are not. All are designed to keep you at ease and in control of your own medical care.

The Right To Confidentiality

Health care is a very private matter. Not only is it extremely personal, but what others know about our health can, and sometimes does, hurt us. For example, there was a time not too many years ago when cancer victims lost their friends, jobs and standing in society due to irrational fears that the disease was somehow contagious.

Doctors and society have long recognized this and thus physicians are duty-bound to keep the details of their patient's health a matter of the strictest confidence and discretion. In fact, it's the law. Doctors cannot be compelled, even in court, to reveal any information given to them by a patient or about what they have observed during the exam or about the diagnosis itself, except under limited and defined circumstances (which we will discuss) or unless the patient consents.

There's a practical side to the issue of confidentiality as well. Doctors know that unless a patient is sure that what is told to the doctor is safe from the gossip mill, there won't be many patients willing to be candid, which in turn would hinder doctors from rendering effective care. This would lead to more illness, reducing the general health of the community as a whole.

Hint: Your right to confidentiality is also binding on the doctor's staff, who may overhear conversations or type reports or read test results. Thus, if one of the doctor's staff tells you about another patient's health, complain to the doctor. After all, that staff member might be telling that other patient all about you.

Few "rights" are absolute, and this one is no exception. The following are three of the more common exceptions to the right of confidentiality:

1. If you sue your doctor for medical malpractice.

Many doctors these days feel as if malpractice lawsuits are turkey shoots to which they have been invited—as the turkeys. However, it often isn't until patients are hip-deep in the litigation that they suddenly realize that some shots are being fired at *them* as well. This "defensive volley" often takes the form of using the patient's own confidential statements or the contents of the patient's own medical chart to disprove the allegations made in the lawsuit. So, if you plan to sue your doctor, also plan to lose your right to confidentiality, at least as it pertains to the allegations in the lawsuit.

2. If your physical or emotional health becomes an issue in a lawsuit.

When you are sued or sue, you lose a great deal of your privacy. If the lawsuit involves your health, your medical records can become fair game. For example, let's say that you have been rear-ended in your car as you waited at a stoplight. You receive injuries to your neck for which you seek medical treatment. You sue for damages. Not only do the medical records of that treatment become an open book, but under some circumstances your past medical history does as well. That's because a common defense in such lawsuits is to prove that your medical problems were not caused by the accident, but already existed (known in legal circles as a "pre-existing condition").

3. If you suffer from what is called a "reportable condition."

In a free society separate rights often come into conflict, forcing society to choose which right shall dominate. When it comes to health, fighting some communicable diseases is viewed as more important than the right of confidentiality. Thus doctors are required by law to report patients who have certain diseases to the state board of health so that action can be taken to prevent the disease's spread.

A classic example of how this works is when a patient is diagnosed as having syphilis. That condition will be reported by the doctor to the appropriate authorities, who will then interview the patient regarding from whom he or she may have picked up the disease and to whom they may have given it. Then these individuals will be contacted, warned they may be suffering from the disease and urged to seek treatment. They will also be interviewed, all toward the end of preventing the spread of the disease.

NOTE: Even in reportable cases, the patient still holds the right to have his or her condition held in confidence from those who do not have a "need to know." For more details on how the system works in your area, ask your doctor or state board of health.

There are over fifty reportable conditions which include the following: Anthrax, Botulism, Gonorrhea, Hepatitis, Cholera, Meningitis, Human Rabies, Rubeola, Syphilis, Trichinosis, Tetanus, Typhoid Fever, Typhus Fever, Whooping Cough, Yellow Fever, and most recently, AIDS.

A Note About AIDS:

There is a major controversy surrounding this dread disease concerning the issue of confidentiality. Most states require that a diagnosis of AIDS be reported. But many do not require that ARC (AIDS Related Complex) be reported, nor do they require that the existence of AIDS antibodies in the bloodstream be reported, even though that condition indicates that the person is infected and can pass the disease on to others. The law in the field is extremely volatile and varies from locality to locality. If you have concerns about your rights to confidentiality with regard to AIDS, be sure to ask your physician in advance of testing, or call the National AIDS Hotline at (800) 342-AIDS.

• The Right To Cleanliness •

Believe it or not, even in this day and age there are doctors who are lazy about their duty to keep their examining rooms clean and antiseptic. (Two members of my own family have witnessed this problem within the last few years.) Unsanitary conditions obviously spread disease, and so part of your job as a "powerful" patient is to look out for signs of uncleanliness and to complain about them when they do appear.

Now, I realize that you can't walk around with a microscope checking for germs and other microorganisms, but you can check to be sure that your doctor meets the following minimum standards of cleanliness.

• The *examining table* should be clean, i.e., not covered with dried liquids (or wet liquids, for that matter). Standard practice is for the table to be covered with fresh tissue paper after each patient. If the tissue paper is wrinkled, speak up.

• Look around the *examining room.* It should be *neat and clean,* with no signs of spilled fluids or equipment lying around. It should also have a clean, antiseptic smell. If you smell any foul odors, complain. After all, when it comes to cleanliness, where there's smoke, there's fire.

• The doctor should *wash his or her hands* in your presence. If your doctor doesn't, don't assume that it was done before he or she entered the room. Just say, "Excuse me, but I have this 'thing' about cleanliness and I didn't see you wash your hands." If your doctor takes offense, you may have learned something about him or her that you definitely need to know.

• The *alcohol in the thermometer jar should cover the entire area* that will come into contact with your body. Alcohol evaporates pretty quickly and it is easy for the level to drop and not be noticed. If you notice this has happened, point it out to the doctor or nurse and make sure the thermometer you use has been sterilized before you put it in your mouth (or anywhere else).

Many doctors now use disposable thermometers or disposable plastic sheaths to cover a nondisposable one. If yours does, make sure it is in its original package before you use it. If your doctor uses a digital thermometer, make sure the mouthpiece is sterilized or is disposable.

• *Syringes and needles should always be of the disposable variety.*

• If your doctor is going to examine a body cavity, he or she *should wear disposable gloves.* This is also true where his or her hands will come into direct contact with body fluids. (The AIDS epidemic being what it is, any medical professional who doesn't wear gloves is either uninformed, lazy or suicidal.)

• *Urine samples* should be collected in *disposable containers.* This is not only for sanitary purposes, but it also protects the specimen from contamination.

• Be sure the *nurse doesn't engage in any unsanitary practices.* A nurse who is assisting in the examination should take the same precautions as the doctor. For example, if a nurse is going to touch any instruments, he or she should also wash his or her hands.

Sometimes it's the "little things" that can make for an unclean condition. For example, my wife was shocked when a nurse blew into the doctor's disposable gloves that were going to be used during the examination. When she complained, the nurse couldn't seem to understand that she had just contaminated what were supposed to be sanitary gloves.

NOTE: Had my wife not exercised patient power by speaking up, she would have been exposed to a very unsanitary condition. Severe infections have been caused by a lot less.

Of course there are many other signs that a doctor does not engage in sanitary practices, from the presence of uncovered waste materials to the doctor having dirty fingernails. The key point to remember is that if you feel that you are being exposed to such a condition you must speak up or you may end up suffering in silence.

• The Right To Dignity •

There are few times in life when we feel more vulnerable than when we are being examined or treated by a doctor. After all, we are literally putting ourselves in the hands of another—which is a little scary under the best of circumstances. Add in the fact that we may not have our clothes on and it's no wonder that some patients become easily embarrassed or intimidated.

Part of your doctor's responsibility to you, the patient, is to minimize this potential discomfort by preserving your dignity. Here's a sample of the treatment you have a right to expect from your doctor.

Draping: Draping is an interesting word which means that you have the right to have your body covered except for the part that must be exposed in order to be examined. Sometimes this is accomplished by issuing you one of those gowns that have a severe draft problem in the rear, while at other times you may be allowed to leave your clothes, or at least your underwear, on during the examination or treatment. And once a procedure is completed, you definitely have the right to cover up again. In other words, at no time should you have to sit around in the nude.

The Presence of a Nurse: Women who are undergoing pelvic or breast examinations have the right, and should insist upon, having a female nurse present, especially if the doctor performing the exam is a man. This way the patient can be assured that she is not in danger of molestation (yes, it *does* happen). This practice also protects doctors from enamored patients or baseless accusations (which also happens).

Privacy: Regardless of whether you are in a doctor's office, an emergency room or a hospital ward, you have the right to have your privacy protected and maintained. This may mean a closed door when undergoing a physical, a drawn bedside curtain in a hospital or a nurse asking visitors to wait outside while you receive treatment. Whatever privacy may mean to you, if you feel like yours is being violated, complain. After all, medical care was not meant to be received in a goldfish bowl.

Hint: If you receive treatment in a "teaching hospital" don't be surprised if you lose some of your privacy, since your case will be used as a teaching example for the doctors of tomorrow. However, if you begin to feel that your hospital bed is becoming Grand Central Station, speak up, since "popularity"and recovery may not go hand-in-hand.

A Clinical Demeanor: The last thing a doctor should do when examining or treating a patient is act in a nonclinical manner. For example, a doctor who sees something he or she doesn't like and says "Uh oh" isn't exactly doing the patient a favor. Nor should the doctor or other treating personnel react to a patient's body or medical condition in any way that would be embarrassing or cause the patient any emotional discomfort whatsoever. (In other words, wolf whistles are definitely out.) That isn't to say that the doctor or nurse shouldn't be friendly and try to put the patient at ease—they just shouldn't get intimate or personal.

There is another aspect of the right to dignity which can be very important to patients and their families alike. And that is the *right to die with dignity.*

Unpleasant as it may be to contemplate, there comes a time in each of our lives when we must, as Shakespeare so artfully put it, "shuffle off this mortal coil." (Although some try to deny the inevitable: Guy Stockwell, the actor, tells a story about sharing a "white knuckle" plane ride with a businessman when the subject of death came up. At one point the man said, "If I die, it won't be in an airplane." Guy chuckled and responded, "What do you mean *if*?" The man gave Guy a horrified stare and refused to talk to him for the rest of the flight.)

While it is true that death cannot ultimately be prevented, it can often be significantly delayed by the miracles of modern medical science. Some of us embrace this new technology while others are repulsed by it, preferring to let nature take its course. This has given rise to serious ethical debates about when and if a patient, or his or her family or doctor, has the right to withdraw life-sustaining treatment when that patient has been diagnosed as having a terminal disease, condition or injury.

It is generally recognized that a patient who is mentally competent has the right, upon giving informed consent—that is, making a decision based on all the information necessary to make an informed and intelligent choice—to have his or her wishes regarding "extraordinary means" to prolong his or her life when the "clock has just about run out of time" carried out. If the decision is to have life prolonged, medical science has the equipment necessary to maintain the functions of the body almost indefinitely. If it is not, there are alternatives, such as the hospice movement, which seek to maintain the comfort and quality of life, while not attempting to prolong its duration. When facing a terminal illness, these matters should be agreed upon ahead of time among the physician, the patient and the family, as should the course of action (or inaction) to be taken.

But what if the fates don't warn us of our impending doom? Say we're hit by a truck and rendered comatose with no hope of recovery. What then? Do we have to rely on our family to read our minds? Should the doctors or the courts be allowed to make the final choice? In many states, the answer is a loud and resounding, *no.*

In those states, we can prepare legal documents ahead of time which leave binding instructions as to how we are to be treated. These documents go under different names — they may be called "Living Wills" or, perhaps "Durable Power of Attorney for Health Care Decisions." But whatever they are called, they permit *you* to be in the driver's seat concerning your own "final curtain."

Hint: These documents are not binding in every state. However, even if they have no legal effect, filling one out will at least inform your family and your doctors about how you wish to be treated.

Hint: The rules concerning Living Wills are also different in each state. Thus, it's a good idea to discuss the matter with your doctor or an attorney ahead of time in order to ensure that you "dot all the I's" and "cross all the T's."

Hint: Fill-in-the-blank type forms are usually available to help you prepare a Living Will. Ask your doctor, attorney or your local medical association how to obtain one in your area.

• The Right To Decide •

The bottom line of health care (and this book) is that when you need medical treatment, the decision as to which way to go and how to get there must ultimately be *yours.* After all, it is *your* body and it is *your* life.

But, you may ask, isn't it your doctor's job to do whatever he or she thinks is best for you? Aren't we patients supposed to give ourselves over to medical professionals and simply let them do their thing? After all, aren't we supposed to trust our doctors?

The answer, of course, is that at some point we must trust our doctors. But that trust should be *earned,* not blindly given. Thus, before a doctor can treat you, with few exceptions, you must give your permission. And this permission must be based on full disclosure to the patient of the potential risks and hoped for benefits of the proposed procedure. In other words, *you have the right to know the pros and cons of each test and each plan of treatment,* and then *you* have the right to make the choice. This concept isn't my idea, but is recognized in law as the twin doctrines of "*Informed Consent*" and "*Informed Refusal*" the key word being *informed.* Let's take a look at how this works. When you feel ill, your doctor's job can be broken down into several parts:

Diagnosis: The first thing your doctor must do is try to find out what is wrong. In order to do so, he or she may have to recommend certain diagnostic tests which will either disclose what the ailment is, or at the very least, tell your doctor what it isn't, since a large part of diagnosis is a "ruling-out process." When it comes to tests, you have the right to give an informed consent or make an informed refusal, since many have potential dangers or side effects. Let's eavesdrop on Dr. I. M. Sketchy, as he explains to his patient, Fraidy Cat, the ups and downs of a proposed (and for our purposes, fictional) diagnostic procedure.

The Wrong Way

Dr. Sketchy:	Fraidy, I want to give you an electroinvasive organoscopy.
Fraidy:	Say, what?!
Dr. Sketchy:	Now don't be alarmed, it's not as bad as it sounds. It's just a simple procedure which will tell me why you have started to graze like a cow.
Fraidy:	Moo!
Dr. Sketchy:	I take that as a yes, so let's get started.

What's wrong with this picture? Fraidy has not been told anything at all. For example, what exactly is an "electroinvasive organoscopy?"

Does it involve any danger? Will it hurt? Will Fraidy have to go to a hospital to have it done? If so, for how long? Are there any potential side effects? Is there another test that can be tried which is safer? How much does it cost? The answers to these and other questions is what a patient must have if he or she is to make an informed consent.

Now let's see how Dr. I. Am Thorough handles the same situation.

The Right Way

Dr. Thorough:	Fraidy, I want to give you an electroinvasive organoscopy.
Fraidy:	What is that?
Dr. Thorough:	It's a procedure whereby we insert a needle into all of your vital organs and give them a mild electric shock. We then read how they react on an x-ray monitor in the hopes of finding out why you have started chewing cud.
Fraidy:	Swell.
Dr. Thorough:	Before you decide, you have the right to know about the side effects. Forty percent of the patients undergoing the procedure feel a tingling throughout their bodies for at least three weeks. The effect is harmless, but it is rather annoying. A few patients suffer permanent deafness caused by the eardrum's adverse reaction to electricity. On the other hand, an accurate diagnosis is

	made in eighty percent of the cases, which is why I recommend the test to you.
Fraidy:	How much does it cost?
Dr. Thorough:	Fifteen hundred dollars, plus the cost of two days' hospitalization. Your health insurance should pay for most of it.
Fraidy:	Are there any alternatives?
Dr. Thorough:	Well, I suppose we could . . . etc.

This conversation should continue until Fraidy Cat has been given all of the information necessary to make an intelligent and informed decision. Thus, if he says, "Let's go for it!" that decision would be made with eyes wide open as to the potential benefits and risks of a procedure, while a "No way, José!" would be made with a full understanding of the potential consequences of refusing the test or procedure.

Treatment: After a diagnosis has been made, a similar process occurs as the doctor and patient work together to decide how the affliction will be treated. Here again, informed consent and informed refusal come into play. For example, if surgery is proposed, the patient should be told the reasons for the surgery, what alternatives exist, what the prognosis is if the patient elects to proceed and what the dangers are, whether from the procedure itself, the anesthesia or potential complications. Similarly, when a doctor suggests treatment by medication, the patient should be told the name of the drug, what it is supposed to do, how often the treatment works and the expected and potential side effects. In all cases a patient should be told what can be expected if he or she refuses treatment.

If doctors *don't* encourage informed consent they expose themselves to malpractice suits if something goes wrong, so you can bet that most make a point of giving you the facts. If yours doesn't, be sure to ask questions. In this way, "the system" has put the ultimate responsibility for your health care in your very own hands—right where it belongs.

Hint: Many medical procedures are complicated and difficult to comprehend. Be sure to ask your doctor to use words you can understand when he or she is discussing these issues with you. You can also ask your doctor if there is any written material you can take home and study before making a decision. After all, most situations don't require instant decisions, and you know what they say, "Act in haste, repent at leisure."

Hint: Never trust a doctor who refuses to answer your questions by saying, "Trust me. I'm a doctor."

The Right To Know What's Going On

Once you have given your informed consent, you then have a right to know what is going to happen in your treatment, step by step. For example, assume that you have agreed to take a certain medication to cure an infection. Your doctor should tell you how long to take the drug, what to look out for in terms of problems or benefits and what foods, drinks or other medications to avoid.

Hint: Always tell your doctor about other drugs you may be taking before he or she prescribes medication. This is important because sometimes a drug that is beneficial when taken alone can prove harmful when taken at the same time as another medication (or alcohol or even certain foods).

I recently saw an example of this in my own family. My brother-in-law takes pills to inhibit seizures. When he had a minor tooth abscess, the dentist prescribed a simple antibiotic. Within a couple of days the two medications had interacted with each other in such a terrible way that we thought he might have suffered a stroke. So you see, even the most common forms of medication can prove dangerous under the wrong circumstances. (By the way, the dentist never asked whether my brother-in-law was taking any other medication. If your doctor or other health professional also forgets, don't be shy, volunteer!)

In the same way, if you are having surgery, your surgeon should lay out for you in simple terms what is going to happen to you, when and what you can expect to experience each step of the way. Let's rejoin Dr. Thorough as he prepares Fraidy Cat for the next day's surgery:

Dr. Thorough: I think it's important that you understand what you will be experiencing tomorrow when we remove that extra stomach which has been causing you to act like a steer.

Fraidy: I don't want to think about it.

Dr. Thorough: I understand, but we have found that patients do better when they know what to expect.

Fraidy: O.K. shoot, er, I mean talk.

Dr. Thorough: In the morning, you'll be given a sedative which will cause you to feel very drowsy. During the surgery, you will be unconscious.

Dr. Thorough: The first thing that you'll notice after the surgery is that you'll feel exhausted. If you feel sick to your stomach, don't be alarmed, that happens all of the time, but try and tell the nurse. (Etc.)

Of course, if you are going to undergo a surgical procedure, or any other form of treatment for that matter, you should receive many more details than provided in this example. However, if you don't, be sure to ask. After all, when it comes to medical care follow in the footsteps of the Boy Scouts. In other words, *Be Prepared.*

The right to understand what is going on with your own body isn't limited to learning the details of proposed treatments. For example, assume that you have been diagnosed as having high blood pressure. You should make a point to learn all you can about the affliction, its potential consequences and the behavior that you and your doctor can decide you should follow to help keep it under control, such as changing your diet.

Hint: Many of the doctors I spoke with tell their patients to learn all they can about their own specific health problems. In that way, not only do their patients become educated consumers, but they become empowered to work as equal partners with their doctors in deciding how to manage their own health care.

PLEASE NOTE that this is not the same as *self-diagnosis,* which is not only foolish, but can be dangerous as well.

Hint: You also have the right to understand all about your "healthy" medical care. As we discussed, part of your primary care physician's duty is to educate you about your health and to tell you what to look out for, medicine-wise, at each stage of your life. Thus, just as a parent would not hesitate to ask his or her pediatrician about what to expect during a child's first year of life, an octogenarian should not be shy about asking for education about their particular health needs. And the same thing applies to those of us in between.

The Right To The Prompt Return Of Test Results

Doctors sometimes seem to forget how nerve-wracking it is to take medical tests and then sit at home waiting to hear the results. I mean talk about losing sleep! I remember a time when a friend had to have a biopsy. Three weeks she waited, assuming that the time delay was caused by concerned technicians double- and triple-checking the test results which had proved to be cancerous. When she could finally not take it any longer, she went to the doctor's office, where her doctor breezily told her that her lump had been nothing but a harmless cyst. The lump she almost put on the doctor's head was anything but harmless!

In order to avoid this form of Chinese water torture, ask your doctor how long it will take for the test results to be ready, and make an appointment then and there to review what the tests will have disclosed. Tests generally can be ready within a few days. Unless your doctor has his or her own lab, this is usually how the system works:

• Your doctor either takes the test and sends the tissue samples (or blood, urine, etc.) to the lab, or sends you directly to the lab to have the tests performed.

• Then the lab performs the analysis. Routine tests are generally processed on a daily basis, while more specialized analysis may be performed once a week or so.

• Special labeling precautions are taken to ensure that one person's specimen is not mixed up with that of another.

• Once the analysis is complete the lab prepares a written report for your doctor, who analyzes what it all means and then passes that information on to you.

Hint: If your tests are not routine as part of a physical but to determine if you may be ill, it's always a good idea to talk with your doctor about the results in person rather than by phone. Phone conversations have a tendency to be impersonal, and if the news is bad, you will want to have the time to ask questions.

Hint: Some tests, such as the one that reads positive for the AIDS antibody, are reviewed by more than one lab and thus take longer to get the results. If in doubt, ask your doctor.

The Right To Be Treated With Respect

When it comes to medical care, too many patients are made to feel like Rodney Dangerfield. Part of patient power is refusing to put up with behavior by doctors or their staff that is insensitive, discourteous or disrespectful. (After all, your business is helping pay the doctor's house payment and the receptionist's salary.)

Respect means different things to different people. Some disrespectful attitudes are simply rude, others, as we shall see, can actually be dangerous to your health.

Staff Courtesy

Telephone Calls: One of the important jobs your doctor's nurse or office staff performs is to protect the physician's time so that he or she can function efficiently. Thus, when you call asking to speak with the doctor, don't be surprised if you are asked the purpose of your call so that the staff member can decide whether your problem is urgent enough to interrupt an examination or conference, or to have the doctor "beeped." This process known as *triaging,* is perfectly fine if it is done with a courteous attitude and in a friendly, businesslike way and if it ends with a promise to have the doctor return your call. What is *not* acceptable is an office member who tells a patient to stop crying, who tells a patient that his or her problem is not important enough to bother the doctor with or who otherwise acts like Nurse Ratched of *One Flew Over The Cuckoo's Nest* fame.

Office Visits: When you arrive in the office you have the right to be greeted promptly and to be told how long your wait to see the doctor will be. (And there's *always* a wait, even for the first patient of the morning.) At no time should the receptionist comment on your prognosis or how successful the outcome of your treatment will be. In fact, the receptionist probably shouldn't comment on your condition at all. Again, if you are ignored or treated unprofessionally in any way, you are not receiving the service you are paying for.

Hint: If you have the misfortune to be confronted by an "attack trained" receptionist, be sure to tell your doctor. More than one doctor has lost good patients because of poor support staff and wondered what went wrong. Besides, if the doctor doesn't care enough about you or your business to see to it that you are treated with respect, then the time probably has come to find another doctor anyway.

Office Policy

In addition to maintaining a courteous and professional staff, the procedures under which the office is operated should be designed to maximize your comfort and convenience. This may be important, because if a doctor has difficulty managing the office, it may tell you something about how that doctor "manages" your health care. Simple things spell r-e-s-p-e-c-t such as:

A "No Smoking" Policy: Smoking is not only bad for smokers, but recent studies indicate it is unhealthful for nonsmokers as well. And since you are in a medical office, it seems that a no smoking policy is the least your doctor can do.

Neat and Clean Waiting Rooms: Visiting doctors is not most people's idea of fun, so the least your doctor can do is make the experience as pleasant as possible by seeing to it that the waiting room is neat and clean and has comfortable chairs. (And hey! How about some magazines published after man first landed on the moon!)

A Short Wait: If there is one thing that doctors are almost universally guilty of, it is forcing their patients to wait "forever" before seeing them, as if your time isn't just as valuable as theirs. (This seeming inability of doctors to stay on schedule is somewhat akin to the inability of most lawyers to return phone calls.) Also, if you are going to have to wait more than fifteen minutes, you have the right to be told as a matter of common respect.

Hint: Since doctors and airline executives seem to go to the same school of time management, it is probably a good idea to call your doctor ahead of time to see if he or she is running late so that you can tell the receptionist that you will be adjusting your schedule accordingly.

Hint: Try to leave yourself plenty of spare time between your doctor's appointment and your next obligation. After all, why risk a diagnosis of hypertension because of a blood pressure reading taken when you are already twenty minutes late to your next appointment?

The Doctor

No Interruptions: When you do get in to see the doctor, you have the right (except in an emergency) to monopolize his or her time. That means no interrupting phone calls, no stepping out of the room to take care of other matters (once you are in conference or are actively being examined) and no "time outs" to say hello to a friend who happens to drop by. To paraphrase a line made famous by Ronald Reagan, you're paying for that "microphone" (in this case, time) and by golly, you should control who gets to use it.

Full Attention: If your doctor seems distracted or pressed for time, he or she may not be giving you the best medical care, which could definitely prove hazardous to your health. Thus if you say, "Give it to me straight Doc, I can take it. How long have I got?" and your doctor replies, "I should never have invested in pork bellies," you may have a bit of a problem.

Treats You as an Equal: Just because a doctor may be more educated than you are or makes more money than you do, doesn't make him or her better and doesn't give him or her the right to treat you with condescension or arrogance. The doctor is there, after all, to *serve*, and if some of us have forgotten that, it's time we were all reminded. Remember, you never have to put up with treatment that makes you feel any less than an equal.

Hint: I was once asked how a guy who drove a Chevy could hope to have an equal relationship with a professional who drove a Mercedes. "Simple," I said, "the guy with the Chevy paid for the Mercedes." I think patients would feel less intimidated if we remembered that.

Is a Good Listener: On occasion, a minority of doctors don't listen to what their patients tell them, or try to trivialize their distress. This can really be dangerous, and while I am not a fan of "doctor horror stories," this one is important enough to pass along.

A medical secretary was about to undergo surgery. As she was being wheeled into the operating room, she suddenly felt a terrible pain which she described as what felt like an elephant sitting on her chest. She told the anesthesiologist, who replied, "Don't be a baby. You're just nervous." When she woke up from surgery, she was in the Intensive Care Unit suffering from a pulmonary embolism.

Sometimes our bodies know more than our doctors. If your doctor doesn't respect what your body is saying, respect yourself enough to find a doctor who will.

The Right To Obtain A Second Opinion

Doctors are people too, and sometimes they make mistakes. The problem is, the consequences of their mistakes can fall awfully hard on us. That's why patients must feel free to get a second—or even a third—opinion if they fear that their doctor's diagnosis of health or illness or his or her recommended course of treatment is in error or misguided.

One way to tell whether you definitely need a second opinion is if your doctor takes offense or appears unduly sensitive to your questions or to the issue of another opinion itself. After all, ego and good medical care do not go hand-in-hand. In fact, if another doctor finds that your first doctor was in error and your first doctor doesn't rejoice, then your health is obviously not the most important item on that doctor's agenda.

Take your time and choose carefully when finding the second doctor. Your best bet is probably to get a certified specialist (or sub-specialist, if appropriate) in the area of concern since you are not looking for a relationship but an expert clinical opinion.

The second doctor should have all of your test results made available since there's no point in undergoing them again. And don't be afraid to have your first doctor discuss your case. After all, the three of you should be a team which works together to solve your health problem.

Beware of a doctor who tries to "steal" you from the physician you have been going to by telling you negative things about the first doctor or by seeming to tell you what you want to hear. That's not to say that you can't decide to stay with the second physician, but if you feel like a piece of fruit about to be picked, the second doctor may have just bought a house at the beach and you may be the mortgage payment.

Once the second opinion has been rendered, make sure it is communicated in writing to the first doctor along with any additional test results, so that you and your doctor can discuss the results and decide where to go from there, even if where you go is back to the second doctor.

Hint: Many insurance companies pay only limited benefits if you fail to obtain a second opinion before non-emergency surgery or hospitalization, while paying full benefits if you do. The difference between having a second opinion and not can literally run into the thousands of dollars. And so, unless you feel obliged to improve your insurance company's profit margin because of all the free calendars they have given you, be sure to check your policy ahead of time.

The Right To Know The Price

Medical care has traditionally been a "fee for service" industry. In other words, patients were billed a specific amount per procedure, as opposed to, say lawyers or plumbers, who might bill based on the "time" it took to perform the service.

Today, the ways in which patients are charged for medical services is beginning to change. For example, Health Maintenance Organizations

(HMOs) have revolutionized the industry by providing health plans where the price of membership pays for substantially all of your health needs (sort of a service contract for medical care). The Medicare DRG system (see chapter 5) has further blurred the "fee for service" concept, as have doctors, notably pediatricians and obstetricians, who charge a fixed fee for a specified period of health services.

Regardless of the way you will be charged for medical services rendered, you have the right to know ahead of time approximately how much a service will cost, how much will be paid by health insurance and when your share of the bill will be due.

Here are some tips to help you deal with this important subject:

• **Ask ahead of time what the procedure will cost in its totality.** It's important to understand that your medical care is frequently fragmented, meaning that different persons or entities have the responsibility for different aspects of your care. Let's take the example of surgery. You will have to pay: the surgeon; the assistant surgeon; the anesthesiologist; the primary care physician who follows your care; the hospital for the use of the facility and for the use of their supplies; and miscellaneous expenses such as lab fees, or in some cases, medical consultant fees or even home nursing care. Thus, the patient who assumes that the total cost of surgery is the surgeon is like the captain of the Titanic who assumed that all there was to that iceberg was what could be seen above the surface. Asking what the *total* cost of your care will be can help you maneuver your financial ship so as to keep it afloat in the fiscal sea.

• **Ask to see a sample bill and have it explained to you.** Sometimes in this age of computerized billing it seems that what you see on the bill is designed to confuse rather than illuminate, so ask your doctor to show you a sample of his or her bill and explain how the system works so that there will be no misunderstanding.

• **Ask whether your doctor will "accept assignment" of your health insurance benefits.** Some doctors make you pay for services as soon as they have been given, forcing you to wait for reimbursement from your insurance company. Others will "accept assignment" which means that they receive payment directly from the insurance company and bill you for the difference. If paying a lump sum fee up front will mean that your family will be eating peanut butter and jelly sandwiches for dinner for the next year, the answer to that question could be important to you.

Hint: If you are on Medicare, ask whether your doctor will accept the fee Medicare rules is reasonable for the service rendered as his or her entire fee, and what your co-payments, if any, will be. The difference in the money you will owe a doctor who accepts the Medicare determination and one who doesn't can be the difference between a comfortable retirement and the poor farm (see Chapter 5).

• **Ask your doctor what he or she will do to help you meet your financial obligations.** Doctors in private practice are business persons and as such they must "market" their services to the general public. Part of this task is to maximize the financial convenience to you, their paying customers. This may come in the form of assisting you with those complicated health insurance forms or it may be accepting a monthly payment plan or credit cards. But whatever it is, if you have special financial considerations, ask your doctor to accommodate you. You will be surprised at how willing he or she may be to help you out. Besides, if *your* doctor won't, there are probably doctors out there who will.

• **If you think there has been an error, speak up.** Doctors should not be treated any differently than any other business concern, and this especially applies if you believe you have been overcharged or if you don't understand your bill. Most doctors will have a bookkeeper who can help you out, but if that doesn't work, go directly to the doctor with your concerns. And whatever you do, don't pay a bill you don't owe.

Hint: Many local medical societies help their member doctors work out patient disputes regarding billing. If your doctor is a member of such an association and you have a billing bone to pick, try giving the medical society a call. After all, mediation beats going to court any day.

The Right Not To Be Abandoned

Once your doctor has accepted you as a patient and has become your doctor, he or she cannot simply terminate that relationship at will. Generally, the relationship can only be terminated in the following ways:

- Voluntary withdrawal by the patient
- The lack of need for further care
- The withdrawal by a doctor after the patient has had the opportunity to find replacement care of equal quality

In other words, if you are ill and in need of treatment and can't pay your bill, your doctor cannot just throw you to the wolves of your affliction, but must maintain your care until you no longer need his or her services or have found a replacement. To do otherwise is to abandon a patient, an act which can be very expensive to the patient's health—and to the doctor's pocketbook when the malpractice verdict hits.

Hint: This applies to doctors only *after* they are retained. A doctor who is not retained can and probably will tell a person who cannot pay for medical services to go to a general hospital, where the words "wait" and "overcrowded" may take on a whole new meaning.

The Right To Copies Of Your File

Many doctors do not encourage their patients to keep copies of their own medical files. Some contend that the patient will not understand what is put in the records. Others assert that such patient "intrusiveness" will create a chilling effect on their doctor's willingness to be honest and candid about the patient on his or her chart. Still others feel as if a patient reviewing his or her own file is akin to a patient looking over the doctor's shoulder.

Well, I say that it is up to the patient and *not* the doctor to determine how deeply involved the patient becomes in his or her own health care. And I say that if patients want to look over their doctor's shoulder, that is their right. Happily, the laws in most states (but amazingly, not all) agree, giving the patient the absolute right to demand copies of his or her own medical records at any time.

So, if you want to keep your own x-rays, ask for a set of copies. If you want a copy of your hospital chart, by all means obtain it. (There will probably be a charge for copying.) In fact, if there is anything you want to see that is contained in your medical records, you should demand the right to do so. After all, the subject of those documents is you.

Hint: There are times when you should obtain your records even if you are not interested in reading them. If you move or if your doctor retires or dies, it's a good idea to get your file so that you can be sure your new doctor will be able to obtain them.

Hint: If you are elderly or have a heart condition, you may want to keep a copy of your EKG (electrocardiogram—a test that charts your heart rhythm on a graph) with you at all times so that any emergency room doctor will be able to see your usual baseline in order to determine if there are any abnormalities.

The Right To Your Doctor's Best Effort

Most doctors are hard-working, dedicated, ethical professionals who pride themselves on their medical skills and their ability to help their patients. Unfortunately, there are a few who either don't know how to care for their patients properly or don't care about them. Those are the ones who can hurt you.

But how does a layperson uneducated in the ways of medicine know if he or she is receiving adequate and proper treatment? It's not easy, but here are a few hints:

• **If your doctor can't answer your questions**—I'm not saying that a doctor has to be able to know instantly the answer to any question you ask. That would be unreasonable. But they should be able to find the answer or at least tell you in pretty explicit detail why there is no answer to give. And so, if you ask your doctor why his or her treatment is the right way to go, and all the doctor says is, "You wouldn't understand," chances are the *doctor* is the one who doesn't understand.

• **If a doctor resents you for wanting to be involved in your own health care**—Most doctors expect their patients to take an active interest in their own medical care. In fact, many I have talked to expressed some astonishment that more of their patients didn't do so. Therefore, if your doctor puts you down or gets angry with you for taking an active interest in what he or she is doing to your body, it could be that that doctor has something to hide.

• **If a doctor resents or resists your obtaining a second opinion**—You and your doctor should want to do whatever it takes to keep or make you well. If that means you have to bring in a second person to confirm a diagnosis or the correctness of a course of treatment, your doctor should encourage your search for truth, not resent it. In fact, a doctor who gets angry at you or tries to talk you out of a second opinion or otherwise acts insecure about your plans to obtain one, may know that there is just cause for his or her insecure feelings.

• **If your doctor talks about his or her own problems rather than yours**—Your doctor has problems just like everybody else, but when they get so bad that he or she talks to you about them instead of why your headaches won't go away, you may have a doctor who is so overwhelmed with his or her own life that the job of protecting yours is playing second fiddle.

• **If you keep suffering setbacks during treatment that were not foreseen by your doctor**—Most treatments have potential side effects which your doctor has a duty to warn you of as a part of your right to give an informed consent. However, if you keep having setbacks which your doctor did not foresee and cannot control, it could be that you have the wrong doctor.

• **If your doctor doesn't want to give you the time of day**—Doctors are in the business of working with people who may be in crisis. Thus, part of their job is dealing with fear and other strong emotions. If you find that your doctor is rude, seems rushed or appears uninterested in what you have to say, it could be that he or she isn't interested, doesn't care or has other matters on his or her mind which are considered more important than your health problems.

• **If your doctor is frequently unavailable**—You want a doctor who is a full-time practitioner, not one who just keeps his or her hand in the business. Thus, if you find that your doctor is on the golf course more than in the office, or is tending to investments far more often than patients, you may have found a doctor who will not be there for you just when you need him or her the most.

• **If your doctor is in poor health**—If your doctor is constantly ill or in poor health, beware. After all, the spirit may be willing, but if the flesh is weak, your doctor may be physically unable to give you his or her best. And when it comes to your health, less than the best just isn't enough.

• **If your sixth sense is screaming, "Beware!"**—Sometimes things go wrong and we sense it long before we can prove that something is amiss. So if your "inner voice" is telling you that your doctor is not giving you all that he or she should, listen to what you are telling yourself. Then talk about your feeling with your doctor or get a second opinion. After all, when it comes to health we usually don't get second chances.

NOTES TO THE CHART

It's always flattering when my patients put me on a pedestal, but that doesn't make it right. The biggest mistake that patients make is treating their doctors like they are divine beings. This inhibits the most important right that a patient has with regard to his or her physician — the right to free and open communication.

One of the things I have noticed about patients is that they are sometimes afraid to ask questions that they believe are "stupid." This is a self-destructive attitude. I can't tell you how many times a patient's hesitant question has shown me that I have not adequately performed my responsibility of informing the patient about his or her illness, either because I failed to get a point across in a way that the patient could understand or, on occasion, because I forgot to mention a topic altogether. For that reason I welcome questions, whether the query is about the treatment I recommend, alternative care or an office policy I might have established. And so does every *good* doctor I know.

Beware of doctors who claim to have an answer for everything. Medical knowledge is far too extensive for any single individual to comprehend every aspect of practice. One of your rights as a patient is to be told by the doctor that he or she *doesn't* know what is going on. In such cases, a second opinion or a referral to a sub-specialist may be recommended, or further diagnostic studies might be ordered to nail down an elusive malady or illness. Whatever the case, *you have the right to know the truth,* your doctor's ego notwithstanding.

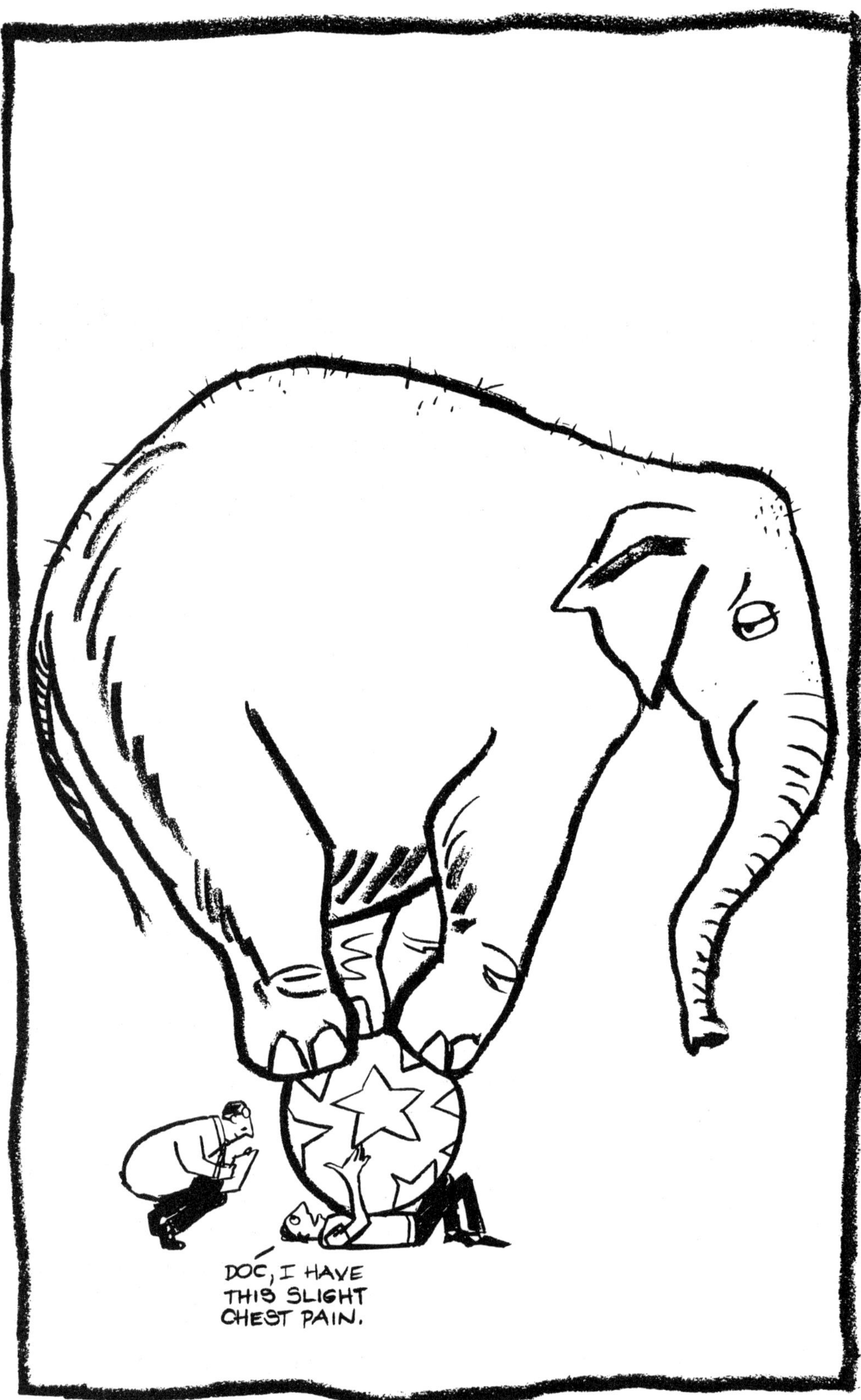
DOC, I HAVE
THIS SLIGHT
CHEST PAIN.

·4·

CHAPTER

Turnabout Is Fair Play

Patient Responsibilities

You and your doctor should be a team joined together to accomplish the purpose of keeping you as healthy as your age, genetic heritage and personal history permit. Like all good teams, each of you has specific duties to perform in order to accomplish the team's goal. When both team members do their respective jobs, the team as a whole is greater than the sum of its parts. When both don't, something gets lost in the equation.

Take Care Of Yourself

At one time in human history, our health was attacked primarily by forces pretty much outside our control. Tuberculosis, polio, smallpox, plague, these and other diseases like measles and even flu, were the killers and maimers that people feared most. The flu epidemics of 1918 killed 548,000 people in this country alone.

Today, thanks to an unrelenting medical war against communicable disease, things have changed. Polio no longer scares millions of children and their parents, as it did me and my folks, with its ugly specter of iron lungs and lifelong physical impairment. Tuberculosis still strikes, but at least with far less frequency in America and with much less devastating an impact, since it is usually curable. And, thankfully, smallpox has been virtually wiped off the face of the earth.

But these killers of the past have given way to a new generation of public health enemies which work unceasingly to shorten life and reduce its quality. I'm talking about heart disease, stroke, cancer, and now AIDS, all of which are striking us down with frightening efficiency.

What is most notable about these killers of today is not that they exist, but that they are in large measure self-induced by our personal habits and the way we live our lives.

• **Smoking:** Smoking is blamed by most health authorities for contributing to a large percentage of heart attacks and for up to eighty-five percent of lung cancers! It is estimated that a thousand deaths a day are directly or indirectly related to smoking. And when you realize that this is a purely voluntary activity, think of the human suffering that could be prevented if the tobacco industry was forced, due to lack of business, to put their tobacco fields to more productive and beneficial use.

• **Excessive Drinking:** Fifty thousand Americans are killed on the nation's highways each year, and over 100,000 are injured in automobile accidents, many of which involve at least one driver who has been drinking. Alcohol abuse also creates significant and sometimes deadly health problems, such as cirrhosis of the liver, not to mention health difficulties created by the stress of lost jobs and broken families that alcohol dependency often leaves in its wake. Smoking and drinking together have been linked in some studies to cancers of the throat and esophagus.

• **Drug Abuse:** A popular rock lyric of the sixties said "Speed kills." It does. So do heroine and cocaine and a host of other drugs. Drug abuse can cause mental and emotional illness. Drug addiction can also lead to crime, which also kills and maims. And if that weren't enough, shared syringe needles lead to AIDS, which leads to death.

• **Diet:** An improper diet can lead to arteriosclerosis (hardening of the arteries), which can result in heart attack or stroke. So can obesity, which also complicates the treatment of diabetes and hypertension.

The point is that much of what kills us and what makes us very sick are things that we can avoid. (Myself included. I weigh more than I should and up until I researched this section of the book, I smoked cigars.) And is it really fair to make ourselves sick and then expect a doctor to be able to undo what perhaps twenty years of self-abuse has created?

Fair or not, it certainly isn't wise. For by living as we do we are very much like Humpty Dumpty, who recklessly decided to sit on that very high wall. And we shouldn't be surprised if our doctors, like "all the kings horses and all the king's men," aren't able to put us back together again.

A Note about AIDS:

While this book is not meant to be used as a medical guide, I believe that something must be said about AIDS.

Today, there is absolutely no reason why somebody who has not already been exposed to AIDS should ever catch the disease. That's because AIDS, like many modern-day ailments, can be avoided by making intelligent choices about our lifestyles:

1. Practice "safe sex." Safe sex is:

a. NO sex (abstinence)

b. Mutual monogamy with an uninfected partner

A simple blood test may tell you with a high degree of certainty whether you or your partner have been exposed.

c. Sex where there is no possible exchange of body fluids, as in old-fashioned necking and petting

2. Practice "less safe" sex, which means using a condom EVERY TIME you make love. THIS IS NOT FOOLPROOF, but it beats unprotected sex and has the side benefit of birth control and protection from other venereal diseases. (Remember, when you go to bed with someone, you are also going to bed with everyone that person has been with since the mid-'70s.)

3. Don't inject drugs. But if you do, use clean, unused sterile needles.

4. When possible, use your own blood for transfusions in surgery. The blood supply is now almost totally free from blood infected with the virus, but not 100 percent clean. So if you have time to store your own blood before undergoing elective surgery, it's a good idea to do so. Besides, it will also reduce your chance of catching hepatitis.

5. Health care workers such as paramedics and nurses should wear surgical gloves when coming into contact with the blood of their patients, since the virus may be able to enter a cut or sore on the skin.

By practicing these measures, you really can prevent the tragedy of AIDS from ever happening to you.

For more information contact the National AIDS Hotline at (800) 342-AIDS, or your local AIDS Project, or ask your doctor.

• Tell The Whole Story •

When you are ill, or even when you are relating your health history to your primary care physician, you must be sure to tell your doctor *the whole story,* even if you find it embarrassing, even if it is criminal in nature, such as if you "do" drugs, and even if you feel it is nobody's business but your own.

Doctors frequently complain that patients withhold important information from them, such as symptoms that the patient doesn't think are important, suspected pregnancies, sexual preference and/or abuse of drugs or alcohol. Patients also seem to frequently "forget" to mention that they are on prescribed medications or that they misuse non-prescription health products such as laxatives. Some patients even withhold the simple fact that they've seen another doctor.

If you have a doctor with whom you don't feel you can be completely candid with about these or other intimate subjects, change doctors. Otherwise, you must be completely open with your doctor about anything that might affect your health. (When in doubt, let your doctor decide whether it's important.) The consequences of doing otherwise can be devastating, like the following.

Failure To Diagnose: Nothing is more frustrating to you or your doctor than when you are not feeling well and your doctor can't identify the problem. Not only does this delay treatment, but it casts a pall over your doctor's expertise as a physician, which weakens the bond of trust you and your doctor have forged together.

When this happens, sometimes the problem is one that requires a referral to a sub-specialist for a second opinion. But sometimes it is caused by "insufficient data." Remember, many of the health problems we suffer from today are caused by the way we live our lives. So don't hesitate to tell your doctor "the truth, the *whole* truth and nothing but the truth." After all, "confession" can be good for your health as well as for your soul.

Misdiagnosis: When health problems arise, they may have an easily identifiable cause. On other occasions, your doctor's job is not so easy and a methodical search is required to solve the "mystery" of why you are ill. At such times your doctor can be compared to Sherlock Holmes, for just as Holmes used clues and deductive reasoning to determine which of several suspects committed a crime, your doctor uses your symptoms and personal medical history to decide which of many possible afflictions is causing your illness or condition.

If you don't tell your doctor the full story or if you actively lie or conceal aspects of your life which may be contributing to your ill health, it's as though someone planted false clues in Sherlock Holmes' path to throw him off the trail. Correction: there is one important difference. The crime

Sherlock Holmes was trying to solve was a creation of *fiction.* Your medical problem may be a matter of fact.

Mistreatment: If your doctor fails to make a diagnosis or actively misdiagnoses your medical problem, the next domino to fall in your search for appropriate health care may be a failure to receive proper treatment.

Receiving the wrong treatment can exact a terrible toll on your health and your future. In the first place, you may lose precious time, which in some situations, perhaps most notoriously with cancer, can be the difference between life and death. Nearly as distressing, you might have strong and powerful drugs administered which in and of themselves create serious side effects that are damaging to your health. If such drugs are given in error, your body's vitality can drop like the stock market did in 1929. At best, you will have lost time feeling ill and wasted money on improper medical care—time that could have been experienced feeling well and having fun, and money that could have been spent paying for it. Life is too short for such folly.

Loss of Doctor Enthusiasm: Doctors, like any of us, work best when they care about what they are doing and are committed to doing it well. In fact, one of the things you should look for in a doctor is this devotion to the healing arts and a deep concern for your individual medical care.

This "fire in the gut" can be doused if your actions or inactions keep your doctor from performing his or her healing function well. Think about it. Imagine how you would feel if you had spent hours sweating over someone's medical problem only to find that your inability to correct the problem was caused by your patient's failure to give "full disclosure." Wouldn't you be tempted to say "Patient, heal thyself" and give a little less the next time you were turned to for help? Well, so might your doctor. Unconsciously perhaps, but after all, it would only be human nature.

Another subject to be candid with your doctor about is money. If you are going to have financial difficulty, your doctor may be able to help out. Here are a few of the ways:

- When it comes to prescribing drugs, there may be more than one way to "medicate" a cat. Generic drugs (non-brand name) are frequently (but not always) equally as effective as their brand name counterparts, yet are usually significantly less expensive. (In fact, Walter Reed Hospital in Washington, D.C., which treats the highest officials in the land, makes extensive use of generic drugs.) So it pays to ask your doctor if a generic prescription will work for you.

• Another way to save money is to ask if the same medicinal treatment can be given in a less convenient form. Today, many pharmaceutical companies are placing great emphasis on convenience in the marketing of their products. For example, some medications that at one time could only be given by injection or by taking medicine several times a day, can now be administered by attaching a "patch" to the skin. Usually, the greater the convenience the higher the cost to you. Thus, if price presents a problem to you, ask your physician if a less convenient and less expensive form of treatment is available (so long as you don't give up any healing benefits).

There are other things your doctor can do, too, like allowing you to make monthly payments or pay by credit card, and by accepting your insurance coverage as payment in full or, perhaps, seeing you a little less frequently if that will not endanger your health. But whatever it may be, you'll never get a chance to enjoy those savings if you don't speak up. After all, there's no board certification available in mind reading.

• Follow Your Doctor's Advice •

Once you and your doctor have agreed upon a course of treatment, listen to what your doctor tells you to do and make a point of following instructions. Also, make a point of asking any questions you have about your treatment before you leave the office, if possible, but in any event, ask them as soon as they pop into your head.

Hint: If your treatment is going to be complicated or you feel as if you will forget your doctor's instructions, have them put in writing. You can also ask your doctor if he or she wouldn't mind if you tape-recorded what you are told to be sure you won't forget.

Take Your Medications As Directed: Your doctor bases the dosage of medication on the amount of the substance that your body can absorb over a period of time, and upon how long the beneficial effect of the drug or chemical lasts. Thus, if you are given a prescription that calls for you to take one pill, four times a day, don't assume that you can take two pills, twice a day. Nor should you assume that taking two pills will produce fifty percent of the hoped-for benefit. Actually, it may not work at all. Similarly, if two medications are prescribed and you only take one, you may be spinning your wheels and paying good money to receive no benefit whatsoever.

Hint: If you "mess up," don't try to correct the error yourself. Call your doctor and "confess" what happened. He or she should know how to get you back on the right path.

You should also take the prescription for as long as you are directed. You know, contrary to what some of us may think, doctors don't direct us to take medication for a certain duration to enrich the pharmacists. They sometimes write prescriptions to prevent a recurrence of a condition once it is beaten, or perhaps, to prevent an associated condition from rearing its ugly and unwanted head. Besides, just because it looks like the coast is clear and you feel "healed," doesn't mean that the enemy isn't lurking in the bushes. So, if you feel as if there is no further need to take your medicine, *ask* before you quit. After all, your doctor is just a phone call away.

Hint: Some medications are given to control chronic conditions which *never* go away. If you are undergoing treatment for such a disease or condition, pay special attention to your medication schedule. Failure to follow instructions can cause your health to go from the frying pan into the fire.

Get Your Rest: Many of us who would never dream of disobeying a doctor's advice about medicine don't think twice about ignoring his or her advice about rest and relaxation. (I'm especially guilty of this.) After all, we've got places to go, people to see, things to do! We're not going to let a little medical condition keep us down!

The fact of the matter is that rest allows the body to do what comes naturally: heal. Healing takes a lot of energy. Thus, if we become active before we are ready, it has the effect of robbing Peter to pay Paul, with our health being Peter. This kind of reckless conduct not only puts us in danger of relapse or reinjury (think of all the sports stars who have really hurt their careers by coming back too soon), but can even cause complications. So don't undo all the good you and your doctor have accomplished together by playing Superman or Superwoman. After all, in real life no one is made of steel.

Do Your Exercises: In medicine, sometimes "no pain" truly is "no gain." Thus, the flip side of the "R & R" coin may be making like Jane Fonda and doing the exercises or physical therapy that our doctor has told us to do, when we are told to do them.

Sometimes proper healing requires that we engage in activity that we would rather not do. This can range from getting out of bed after surgery to undergoing a rigorous course of physical therapy.

Case in point: A friend recently injured her shoulder in a ski accident. No, injured isn't the right word. What she did was *annihilate* it. The only way she could regain full use of her arm was to engage in grueling, painful exercises, which she did religiously despite the fact she was under deadline to write a book. In other words, her health came first, even though it hurt and created a major inconvenience in her professional life. Months later, her shoulder is now fine and her writing project is completed. But had she not had the moxie to make time for the pain, her arm might have been disabled for the rest of her life.

Change Your Lifestyle: Sometimes it seems that all our doctors do is nag, nag, nag. "Quit smoking." "Lose twenty pounds." "Reduce your level of stress." It's enough to really tick a patient off! But the next time you start to get mad, remember: they aren't nagging for their health, but for *yours.*

Don't Wait Until The Last Minute

Doctors work hard for you five days a week (all right, so maybe it's four) and, like most of us, look forward to the time they can spend with their families on weekends. (Many doctors work weekends too, handling emergencies and following patients who may be hospitalized.) That's why doctors hate "Friday Night Specials." These are the patients who get sick on Tuesday and then wait until Friday afternoon to demand that their doctor squeeze them in. This practice is not only aggravating for your doctor (except in urgent cases—after all, if you're sick, you're sick) but has inherent disadvantages for you:

• Your doctor may not be able to squeeze you in. Then you will be caught between a rock and a hard place—required to take a trip to the emergency room, which is time-consuming and expensive, or be forced to "grin and bear it" until your physician can see you at the beginning of the week.

• Even if your doctor *does* agree to see you, labs will not be nearly as understanding since they operate only during normal business hours. Thus, if you wait until the last minute, testing may be hard to come by, or if the test is highly specialized, it may not be available at all. And even if you do find a lab which will accommodate you, your test will be peformed on an overtime basis, and it doesn't take a Ph.D. in economics to tell you what that means.

• Since tests, or at least their results, may not be immediately available, on occasion your doctor may have to have you hospitalized if you are very ill, just to be safe. And, since most hospitals run on reduced staffing during weekends, treatment may have to be delayed until Monday (unless, of course, your condition is very urgent or life-threatening). In short, Friday Night Specials bring with them a tremendous potential for inconvenience, expense, discomfort and potentially health-impairing delay.

All of this doesn't mean that you should sacrifice yourself to protect your doctor's home life. Your doctor realizes that, like a police officer, he or she is never really off-duty, so if you feel you might be seriously ill, by all means, call! Your doctor will tell you if the problem can wait. Just don't put off seeking treatment you need today until next Friday at 5:00 P.M.

Don't Accept Your Friend's Diagnosis

I think that it is safe to say that all of us have "played doctor" at one time or another. No, I'm not talking about "The Birds and the Bees 101," but the tendency of most of us to tell our friends what's wrong with them, or to listen to what our friends say is wrong with us.

This is a mistake. First, similar symptoms can be caused by different conditions. After all, everyone is different. So, just because your friend's daughter had a cough that was diagnosed as a mild bronchitis doesn't mean that your son's cough means he has it too. Second, as we will discuss in more detail in Chapter 6, a proper diagnosis will probably not be made on symptoms alone, but upon a combination of other factors including history, tests and an examination. After all, doctors take a big chunk out of their lives to learn the art of proper diagnosis, so it is highly unlikely that you or your friends can do a better job.

The dangers of listening to or giving "lay" medical advice are obvious. For example, necessary and proper treatment might be delayed in favor of a folk remedy or because a serious condition has been "diagnosed" by Cousin Martha as being "nothing to worry about." Or, you may be needlessly alarmed when your Uncle Art tells you that your athlete's foot is really preambulatory gangrene. However, the most common problems are caused when some people take their well-meaning friend's advice beyond mere diagnosis to the point where they actually take someone else's medication. This is dangerous folly because:

- Some seemingly harmless medicines can actually do grave harm. A typical example are cough medicines with decongestants, which can aggravate high blood pressure.

- As we have already seen, the new medicine you are given can react with a medicine you are already taking to counteract its medicinal value and render both medications ineffective or even create a toxic condition that can seriously endanger your health.

- It may be the wrong medicine for your condition.

- The medicine may serve to mask your symptoms, thus delaying your trip to your doctor and your receipt of appropriate care.

Even if the medicine is the correct one, you won't know the right amount to take since dosage is frequently determined by factors such as height, weight, age, general health, blood test results and seriousness of condition. And since we are like snowflakes in that no two of us are ever exactly alike, the chances of taking the wrong dosage are pretty high—which means that the chances of even the right medicine doing you much good are pretty low.

• Be Prepared •

Your doctor's ability to assist you in caring for your health is in large part dependent on your ability to provide him or her with all of the information needed to do a thorough and competent job. That means you must make a point of compiling all of the data and gathering all of the facts that your doctor will need *before* you attend your appointment.

> **Hint:** Make a point of asking the doctor ahead of time what you should bring with you to your conference or examination so that you and he or she can hit the ground running.

The following is a list of the things your doctor will want to have on file (other than the deed to your house):

• A complete list of medications you take including the *name* of the medicine, the *dosage*, the number of *times* it is taken per day and its *purpose*. The following is a scenario that happens in doctors' offices every day and which you as a powerful patient will never allow to happen to you:

Doctor:	Are you taking any medicine?
Patient:	Yes, I'm taking blood pressure pills.
Doctor:	What is the name of the medicine?
Patient:	I'm sorry, I forgot. They're blue capsules, though. Does that help?
Doctor:	I'm afraid not. I'm sorry, but I can't write you a prescription until I know what medicine you are taking. Is there someone at home we can call?
Patient:	Just Fluffy, my cat.
Doctor:	Then I'm afraid you will have to go home and call me. Then I'll call your pharmacy this evening with the prescription.
Patient:	But they close at five!
Doctor:	I'll call it in tomorrow, then. I'm sorry, it's the best I can do.

The job ultimately will get done, but look at all the wheel spinning!

• The names, addresses and phone numbers of the physicians you have had *over the years*. This can be important when a doctor compiles your medical history, which consists not only of what ailed you, but what was done about it and when it was done. The simple truth is that as time passes, many of us forget this information and your doctor will need a source to call upon to fill in the gaps. Also keep a list of all *hospitals* you've been admitted to.

• A copy of all of your *medical records* in your possession. As we discussed in the last chapter, you should keep copies of all of your own medical records. An important reason for this is so that they may be immediately available to any subsequent physician who needs to know the details of your medical history. Remember, once you cease to be an active patient, your former doctor will store your records in his or her inactive files which might not be immediately available. Besides, doctors have been known to move or die, making your files that much harder to obtain. By keeping copies of the records yourself, think of the time and effort that might be saved when saving time and effort may be really important to you.

• *Insurance records* should be on file and kept up to date so that there are no delays in your treatment and no delays in your doctor's compensation. After all, your doc isn't in practice for his or her health, but for *yours.*

• Have a *translator* available if you don't speak English well and your doctor or his or her staff, doesn't speak your language fluently. After all, if you and your doctor don't speak the same language, it will be awfully hard to communicate.

Hint: You should also make a point of writing down what you need to discuss with your doctor ahead of time. This may include a list of symptoms, questions you want to ask, or the information you have been asked to supply. Remember, what you forget to tell your doctor can hurt you.

Be Specific About Your Ailments

When you are trying to tell your doctor how you feel, the more specific you are, the better your doctor will be able to zero in on the problem. The language you use isn't important. No one expects you to be able to throw words around like, "radiating pain," or "occipital lobe." Just make a point of trying to be as descriptive as you can when telling your doctor "what hurts."

For example, try not to be like this patient, who forces his doctor to play "Guess My Symptom."

Doctor: What seems to be the problem?

Patient: My chest hurts.

Doctor: Please describe the pain for me.

Patient: It's bad, okay?

Doctor: Try to be more specific.

Patient: How can I be more specific? Read my lips—my chest hurts. Am I having a heart attack?

Doctor: I don't know yet. Is the pain sharp? Dull? Does

it feel like someone is sitting on you?

Patient: Yea, like an elephant decided I'm his easy chair.

Doctor: Does any other part of your body hurt?

Patient: Yes.

Doctor: What part?

Patient: My arm.

Doctor: Which arm?

Patient: My left arm.

A better way to handle the situation by the patient would be:

Patient: Doc, my chest hurts. It's a crushing pain like someone was sitting on my chest. My left arm hurts real bad too. Am I having a heart attack?

See how a brief but descriptive summary saves time and aggravation? Also try not to be like Joannie Irrelevant:

Doctor: What seems to be the problem?

Joannie: I was on my way to my sister's house when I saw this pair of shoes in a store window that would match my new plaid skirt perfectly. I knew my sister would be mad if I was late, but I just had to . . .

Doctor: Excuse me for interrupting, but what is the problem?

Joannie: I'm trying to tell you. I went in the store and I asked how much the shoes in the window were. And I couldn't believe how rude that salesman was. Here a paying customer wants help and he won't get off the phone.

Doctor: Please, just tell me why you are here.

Joannie: I'm getting to that. I got so mad that I began to demand to speak to the manager, and that's when I got dizzy.

Doctor: I see. Please try to be a little more descriptive. Did the room spin? Did you faint?

Joannie: I sure felt faint. And do you think that salesman even cared?

Doctor: Did you require assistance?

Joannie: Well, I had to sit down.

(Joannie was heard complaining on the way out that the doctor wasn't a very good listener.)

Here's how Joannie should have discussed her problem:

Joannie: I was having an argument with a shoe salesman when I suddenly felt faint and had to sit down.

This simple sentence told the doctor all that the first conversation did, thus allowing the two of them to get right to other matters at hand, such as whether Joannie suffered any pain or whether she had ever fainted before.

In summary, when you are talking to your doctor, try to be as specific and to the point as you can be. In that way your doctor's job will be made easier and he or she will be able to get to the important task of making you well that much faster.

Tell Your Doctor How You Feel

Part of exercising patient power is giving your doctor the simple courtesy of telling him or her how you feel, both physically and about the way you perceive you are being treated as a human being (one who is paying the bills at that).

On a physical level, your doctor simply must know how a course of treatment is working out. Your doctor doesn't want a "yes patient" any more than you want a doctor who will only tell you what you want to hear. So if the medicine you were given gives you gas, say so. If you are feeling better, let your doctor know. If you have a feeling that "something is rotten in Denmark," speak up, even if you can't put your finger on exactly what is disturbing you. In short, *communicate.* Your doctor *wants to know.*

You should also make a point of telling your doctor if you are satisfied with the way you are treated as a patient. If your doctor's staff has impressed you, give them a boost with their boss. If not, spill the beans. After all, your doctor's business is serving people, and if there is a glitch in the system, he or she has a right to know. Besides, telling your doctor is a lot easier on your nerves and pocketbook than changing doctors because you can't stomach the staff.

This advice applies double to matters directly concerning the doctor/patient relationship. Too many of us are in awe of doctors and tend to treat them with kid gloves rather than speak the truth and let the chips fall where they may. Such timidity isn't doing anyone a favor. Remember, your doctor is not a medium or a trance channeler. He or she can't solve a problem unless it is brought to his or her attention. So, if you are unhappy with your doctor for any reason, schedule a meeting to clear the air. I'll bet that you'll find your doctor will be anxious to resolve the difficulty. And if not, well, it's better to learn that your doctor doesn't care about your business sooner rather than later. In any event, you'll sleep better at night once the problem is out in the open.

A corollary to speaking your mind is showing appreciation. We have become so used to medical miracles and scientific breakthroughs that we tend to forget how hard our doctors worked to learn the healing arts, and how hard they must continue to work to keep current on the latest techniques. So when your doctor "does good," let him or her know how grateful you are and how much better you feel. And when it comes to expressing appreciation, try to walk the extra mile. After all, a thank-you card, a box of candy or maybe even a plant to spruce up the waiting room are a small price to pay to give your doctor that special feeling that comes with a job well done. Besides, the next time you need help, you can bet your doctor will attack the problem with a little extra gusto, which ultimately benefits you.

Be Considerate Of Your Doctor's Time

Courtesy, respect, consideration — we want our doctors to give us all of these. Yet some of us forget that life is a two-way street where what we sow, we reap. Thus, just as you have the right to expect your doctor to be considerate of your time, so should you be considerate of your doctor's.

When you think about it, this patient responsibility really isn't very tough. Just follow these simple rules.

• **Be on time for your appointment and call if you are going to be late.** Remember, you are not your doctor's only patient. When you cause a twenty-minute delay, you are not just inconveniencing your doctor, but every other patient he or she will be seeing during the day. So do your part to stamp out the insidious scourge of *doctor delayitis;* be punctual.

• **Restrict your appointment to the purpose for which it was set.** One of the things your doctor learns very early in his or her career is the importance of budgeting time. Thus, when you call for an appointment, you will be asked its purpose and enough time will be set aside in the doctor's day to accomplish that specific task. The same thing happens with other patients as your doctor puts his or her daily calendar together in such a way as to maximize convenience and efficiency, while accomplishing all that must be done during the day.

Thus, an hour-and-a-half exam might be followed by two fifteen-minute consultations, with a visit to a patient in the hospital coming next and then lunch with the hospital chief of staff. If you are one of the fifteen-minute consultations and try to bring up matters that were not originally scheduled, you put your doctor in the awkward position of either disappointing you, or messing up his or her whole day. So be polite. If you need more time with your doctor, call ahead and rearrange your appointment (except, of course in emergencies). Your doctor's goodwill is too valuable an asset to waste.

• **Cancel appointments you cannot keep.** If you find that you cannot keep an appointment with your doctor, call and cancel at the earliest possible moment. Not only will that assist your doctor, but it could prove important to another of your doctor's patients who may have an urgent concern that needs to be "squeezed in." Besides, imagine how you would feel if your doctor just didn't show up. You'd think he or she was an inconsiderate creep, right? Well, that's just how your doctor will feel about you.

• **Be prepared to deal with the purpose of your appointment.** As stated previously, when you come to your doctor's office, be prepared to deal with the matters at hand. In that way a thirty-minute consultation won't end up taking an hour, leaving other appointments devastated in its wake.

Have Reasonable Expectations

We expect an awful lot of our doctors. Good bedside manners, twenty-four-hour-a-day availability, and a patient recovery rate of nearly 100 percent (except for those patients over 100 years old, where we permit an eighty-five percent recovery rate).

Yet, in truth, doctors are only human and medicine is at best an imprecise science. Thus, while it is easy to get spoiled by medicine's daily successes, it is also unfair to expect continuous "miracles." Here are a few of the things doctors have asked me to tell you about this topic:

• **Don't be angry if it takes more than one visit to reach a diagnosis.** Medicine is frequently as much a "ruling out" process as it is anything else, and thus it may take several office visits or tests to zero in on what the true culprit is. So be a *patient* patient. Realize that your body isn't a computer which will produce results at the push of a button.

Of course this doesn't mean that you have to have the patience of Job. After all, your doctor isn't The Almighty carrying out a perfect plan. So if you haven't found relief within a reasonable time, ask your doctor what the problem is and why it is taking so long to treat. You may find that it's time to see a sub-specialist.

• **Don't expect instant cures.** Your body isn't like an automobile engine which, when given a tune-up, is instantly made as good as new. While it is true that our bodies have amazing restorative powers, they do take time to operate. And since the role of medicine, in actuality, is to assist your body with the job of healing rather than doing the job itself, we should not get angry when we don't receive instantaneous results.

That is not to say that we should not question our doctors if we don't see evidence of progress. Of course we should. And when in doubt, we should not hesitate to get a second opinion. But we should also recognize that healing frequently occurs bit by precious bit, and that your doctor may not be able to speed up the process.

Hint: Your doctor should, however, be able to give you a rough estimate of how long the process is expected to take, and should take action if that timetable doesn't come through. And by the way, if a doctor responds to your request for a time estimate with the words, "These things take time," be sure to ask the key question. *"How Much?"*

• **Realize that a 100 percent cure is not always possible.** The unfortunate truth of life is that our bodies eventually wear out. This can appear to occur "suddenly," as with an unexpected massive coronary, but in reality, our bodies break down slowly over a period of time. Sometimes, an illness strikes or an injury occurs which cannot be completely reversed.

If your doctor tells you this has happened to you, by all means, get a second opinion but don't take your frustrations out on your physician. After all, he or she didn't make the rules.

• **Don't expect your doctor to say what you want to hear.** Your doctor is not in the business of making you happy, but of giving you the straight scoop about your physical health and trying to make or keep you well. Sometimes this means telling you things you'd rather not hear, such as that you had better lose weight or that you or a loved one has a terminal illness or, perhaps, that the baby you had been planning on having is just not in the cards. Your doctor doesn't enjoy this part of the practice any more than you do, so do yourself and your doctor a favor. Don't hate the messenger because you hate the message.

Pay Your Doctor

Last but not least, pay your doctor and cooperate in the processing of insurance forms so that he or she can reap the financial benefits of the services that he or she has rendered.

It is also important for each of us to remember that a doctor in private practice is in business. He or she has a payroll to meet, office rent or mortgage payments to pay and equipment to purchase or lease. Overhead usually amounts to between thirty and fifty percent of a doctor's gross earnings, most of which is directed toward providing comfortable facilities and a well-trained staff, all of which helps your doctor provide you with the best medical care possible.

NOTES TO THE CHART

Doctors are trained to diagnose and treat. That purpose is the ultimate goal behind four years of college, four years of medical school, internship and then, residency. Thus, nothing is as frustrating to a physician as when, despite all of his or her training, a proper diagnosis cannot be made.

On occasion, a proper diagnosis can only be obtained after a methodical search for the cause of the affliction. We usually order tests to rule "in" or "out" suspected causes of symptoms. These tests do not always prove fruitful. At such times, we may have to wait a few days for the condition to establish "markers" which upon being read will permit a proper diagnosis. This period of testing and waiting and testing can really fray nerves.

At such frustrating times, don't take your anger out on your doctor, but try to be patient and work *with* your physician by being totally forthcoming and by keeping track of your symptoms with meticulous detail. Sometimes a little extra effort on the part of the patient is what it takes to break the diagnosis logjam.

If you have been successfully diagnosed and treated by a sub-specialist, don't overlook the contribution of your primary care physician whose work probably made that success story possible. Remember before the sub-specialist ever saw you, your primary care physician had already significantly narrowed the field of possible ailments making the sub-specialist's task that much easier. So when you thank the sub-specialist for making you feel better, also thank your PCP for paving the way.

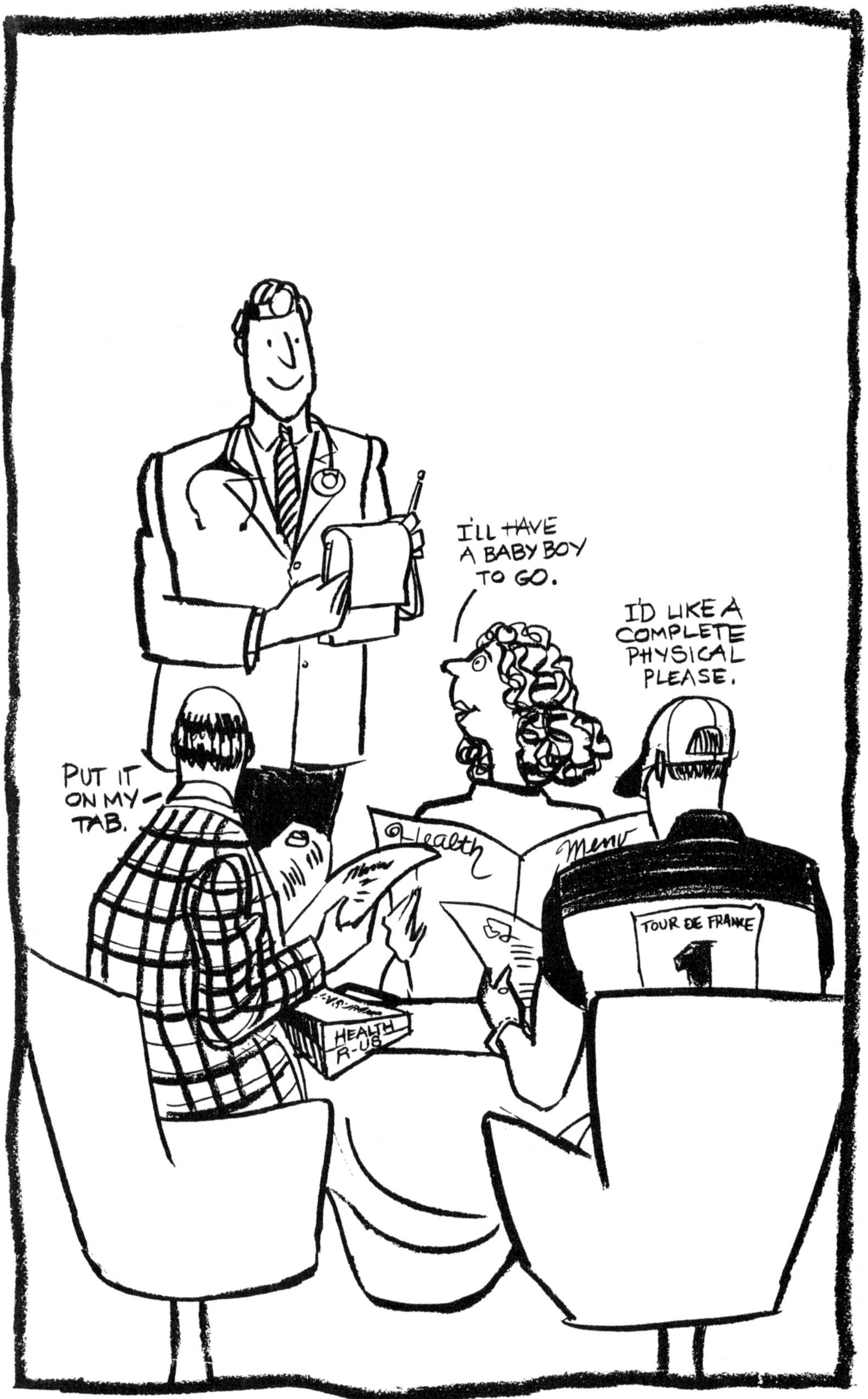
I'LL HAVE A BABY BOY TO GO.
I'D LIKE A COMPLETE PHYSICAL PLEASE.
PUT IT ON MY TAB.
Health
Menu
TOUR DE FRANCE
HEALTH R-US

·5·

CHAPTER

Put It On Their Tab

The Importance Of Health Insurance

Once upon a time in Healthcare Land, there was a doctor, a patient and a chicken. The doctor treated the patient, the patient gave the doctor the chicken and everything was over except for the making of the dumplings. The system was simple, it worked and, of course, over time it was drastically changed.

A new and exciting friend of the people (and the chicken) was created called health insurance. Oh, at first, this too worked simply enough. Rather than giving the doctor your chicken, you gave him or her your health insurance card and your health insurance company paid the doctor for you. Of course you had to pay for your health insurance card, but the peace of mind that came with knowing that the chickens in your coop were safe made the payments all worthwhile.

And then, an ill wind blew into Healthcare Land in the form of rising prices. The doctor who at one time would have been satisfied with the one chicken, now charged the price of the whole farm for his or services. As a result, health insurance premiums skyrocketed and there was ill will and uneasiness in the land.

There then arose among the people a hue and cry for health care reform and cost containment. The purveyors of health insurance responded by offering a plethora of new and more varied health plans, all slickly marketed by the three-piece-suited legions from a place called Madison Avenue. Soon, people didn't know what they were buying. The scent of money was in the air and confusion reigned supreme.

During all this, the cost of medical care was also increasing. Today medical care is very, very expensive. Special care in a hospital can run over $700 a day, and that doesn't include doctors' fees, medical supplies or the cost of medications. The cost of ordinary care is enough to make one's heart skip a beat as well, costing in many instances hundreds of dollars for examinations and lab tests alone.

All of this means that unless you are a Rockefeller, health insurance has become a virtual necessity of life. But which health insurance plan should you take? With so many different types of insurance polices on the market, each offering different costs and benefits, how is one to decide?

The answer, in two words, is comparison shopping. Look over the different plans. See what each charges and what each gives back by way of benefits. Then select the plan which you believe has the best combination of *affordability, reliability, convenience* and *protection* to suit your particular needs.

Monsieur Et Madame, Your Health Plan Menu

~ *The Meat And Potatoes Entrées* ~

When most people think of health insurance, they think of "traditional" or "conventional" plans that pay them or their doctor for services as they are rendered. These types of policies generally come in two distinct types: the indemnity plan and the fee-for-service plan.

The Indemnity Plan is probably the easiest to understand. Simply put, you receive a lump sum benefit, say $200, for each covered day you spend in the hospital. Unfortunately, the benefits you receive are usually far less than the obligation owed, but I suppose it beats not receiving *any* benefits at all.

The Fee-For-Service Plan is far more common, and as we shall see, far more complicated. Under this type of policy, you or your doctor submit bills to the insurance plan setting forth the procedures performed or the dates of hospitalization, and the insurance company pays the portion it is obliged to pay under the policy.

Of course, if matters were that simple, this chapter would never have appeared in this book. Unfortunately, as we will discuss, even conventional policies have become very complicated contracts, indeed.

The following is a nuts and bolts breakdown of how these insurance plans operate. Please note that every policy does not necessarily have each of the following services covered. Check yours or the one you may be thinking of obtaining to see which benefits you are covered by.

Hospitalization

This coverage protects you, as the name implies, when you are hospitalized. The following is what is typically covered under this type of policy:

- A semi-private hospital room and bed
- Routine nursing care (and bedpan service)
- Food (such as it is)
- Use of the operating room, when appropriate
- Minor medical supplies
- Lab tests and x-rays
- Doctors' bills incurred as a result of surgery or hospitalization
- Outpatient care if connected with surgery or an accident that caused the hospitalization

Things To Look Out For

When deciding which policy to choose, or when evaluating whether you need better coverage, find the answers to these questions.

How much of the total price is covered? The best policies cover 100 percent, others cover less or pay on an indemnity basis.

How long does coverage last? Most policies set a time limit for payment of benefits, typically 120 days. Obviously, the longer the protection lasts, the better it is for you.

Is there a wait before benefits begin? Happily, most hospitalizations are not nearly enough to exhaust insurance benefits. A bigger problem exists with policies that force you to be hospitalized for a certain number of days *before* payments begin. Thus, if your policy pays "after the first five days of covered services," and you are hospitalized for seven days, your plan pays for two days.

What is excluded? Like most insurance programs, hospitalization coverage usually sets forth certain "exclusions," which are *not* covered under the policy. My policy, for example, excludes:

• Hospitalizations caused by injuries I might incur in the course of my employment. (And, as we all know, writing is a dangerous profession. I could get my finger stuck in the keyboard of my word processor or develop writer's cramp or even get a paper cut!)

• Hospitalization for diagnostic studies. This means that my policy does *not* cover procedures which must be performed in a hospital, such as an angiogram, during which a tube is inserted into an artery to see if it is clogged up (arterial sclerosis), a condition that can lead to a heart attack.

• Treatment rendered in government hospitals, such as Veterans Hospitals

• Hospitalization for convalescent care

• Hospitalization for self-inflicted injuries or attempted suicide

• Diseases or injuries I might receive as a result of a declared or an undeclared war. (Of course, if we ever have a war there might not *be* a hospital to go to. Do you think they'd give me a partial refund?)

• Outpatient care rendered in other than accidental emergencies

Are pre-existing conditions covered? Of course, insurance executives would love to be able to collect premiums and not be forced to pay benefits. Luckily, they can't get away with that (not for lack of trying), but they can exclude from covered benefits hospitalizations caused by a condition that pre-dates the policy. So, if you have had a previous illness, check into this aspect of coverage thoroughly before you sign your John Hancock.

Hint: One of the benefits of "group coverage" (i.e.,policies offered to specifically identified groups, such as unions or employees of a corporation) over individual policies (i.e., one you buy as an individual) is that pre-existing conditions are frequently *not* excluded, or are included after a defined waiting period. Thus, if a pre-existing condition is a problem for you, investigate whether you qualify for a group plan that will protect you more fully.

Is specialty care covered? By "specialty care" I mean the big ticket items such as the intensive care unit or the coronary care unit, which can run upwards of $700 to $1,000 a day, and is steadily increasing. (Which means that finding out you weren't covered when you thought you were can put you right back into the specialty unit you couldn't afford to pay for the first time.)

Am I fully covered in all hospitals? Some insurance companies contract with certain hospitals wherein the insurance company agrees to "encourage" their beneficiaries to seek medical care in the hospital, in return for which the hospital gives the insurance company a discount on the fees charged. These hospitals are called "contracting facilities." All other hospitals are called "non-contracting facilities." (Clever, no?) These companies "encourage" their beneficiaries to attend contracting facilities by paying a *lower* percentage of the bill in non-contracting facilities. Thus, by being subjected to a simple pain/pleasure principle, you are pushed in the direction that your insurance company wants you to go.

Can the policy be renewed? If the policy is one that does not guarantee your right to renew, be very careful. After all, if you become very ill and use your benefits under a policy in which the company can cancel you, guess who's going to get a letter in the mail expressing the company's "sincere regrets?" And once you've been canceled by Company A, guess who won't be able to obtain a policy from Company B because of the pre-existing condition exclusion? Ain't insurance fun?

Of course, each policy is different, so read yours carefully to see if there are any rattlesnakes lying around in the bushes waiting to be stepped on, or ask your insurance agent or plan administrator to explain fully your policy to you in terms you can understand.

Major Medical

Major medical plans fill in many of the gaps in health care protection which are not covered by basic hospitalization coverage. The major purpose of major medical benefits is to provide protection during major illnesses or prolonged treatment of injuries or other medical conditions. Major medical policies generally have three distinct features:

• **High maximum benefits:** This means that your policy will pay for treatment up to a very high level, such as in my health policy, which will pay up to $250,000 per year.

• **Deductibility clause:** Most policies have a deductibility clause, which can vary from policy to policy. The customary policy provides for a specific deduction to be paid by the beneficiary, say $200, before any benefits are paid. This type of deductibility clause is usually called a *standard deduction.* Some policies provide for what is called *first dollar coverage,* which means that there is no deduction. It's a nice policy if you can get it, but as you can imagine, it's usually very expensive to obtain. Finally, there is a new type of deductibility clause which provides first dollar coverage, but for only a percentage of the cost, typically 50 percent. If you had this type of policy and incurred a medical bill of $500, you'd pay $250 and your insurance company would pay $250.

Hint: Most companies offer plans with different deductibility clauses, where the higher the deductible, the lower the premium (the cost of the policy). If the size of the premium is an issue in your life, try getting a higher deductible. In that way you'll be able to buy your groceries, and you will probably be able to find a physician who will allow you to pay your portion of the bill in monthly payments, while you still have protection against serious illness.

• **Co-payment clause:** Most policies require their beneficiaries to pay a portion of covered medical expenses, most commonly 20 percent, with the insurance company picking up 80 percent. There is also usually a "stop loss" cap, say after the patient has paid $3,500, after which the company picks up 100 percent of the cost for the duration of the year, after which the deductibility and co-payment provisions are reinstated for the next year. As with deductibility clauses, you can obtain less expensive premiums if you increase your percentage of responsibility for covered expenses.

Things To Look Out For

What is excluded under the policy? As with hospitalization insurance, a careful review of exclusions is essential to avoid an unpleasant and expensive surprise. For example, many people are not aware that some policies exclude:

- Maternity benefits for healthy normal deliveries
- Physical exams and other preventive medical procedures
- Pre-existing conditions
- Routine pediatric care
- Expenses that the plan does not consider "*customary and reasonable*"

Hint: Most policies carry a provision that states that their obligation to pay is limited to a percentage of the medical fees that are "customary and reasonable" in your locality. That means that they may not pay a percentage of the *actual fee* that is charged (which is usually higher), thus increasing your co-payment obligation. Talk to your doctor in advance about this issue to see if he or she will take what the insurance company determines is customary and reasonable as the actual fee.

Hint: Some policies have provisions that state if you go to physicians who are members of the health plan, those physicians will take the insurance benefit as payment in full. More on that later.

How does the deductibility clause work? Some companies kick in the deductible for each claim while others apply the deductible to a benefit period, usually one year. Obviously, the former has the potential to be much more costly if you have a series of health problems, while the latter will probably be more expensive to obtain.

Is there an extension clause in the event you are disabled? Many policies provide for an automatic extension of benefits for a specified period of time in the event the beneficiary becomes disabled. This provision is obviously a helpful one, especially if you have to "earn" your benefits by working, in that it will permit you extra time to get back on your feet in the event of a major injury or illness.

Is home care provided for in the policy? With insurance companies becoming less and less willing to pay for hospitalizations, it becomes more and more important that your policy pay for home nursing care as you recover from your illness or injury.

Does the policy have a guaranteed renewability clause? What applies to hospitalization goes double for major medical.

What is the maximum you will have to pay per year? An important part of choosing or evaluating a health insurance policy is determining what the worst case financial scenario is regarding a serious illness. To do that, add the deductible to the maximum co-payment and your total is your worst case scenario (unless your doctor won't accept your insurance company's determination of usual and reasonable charges).

Hint: If you are the beneficiary of more than one health policy, your insurance companies should *coordinate their benefits* on your behalf, which may protect you from most out of pocket expenses. For further details ask your agent or health plan administrator.

How are you updated on your benefit status? As you can see, health insurance is a complicated field and some people find it difficult to keep current on matters such as how much co-payment they may still owe or what has been paid and to whom. Thus, your insurance company should provide you with a status report each time you make a claim that explains what services were paid for, to whom, and the amount, if any, that is still owed as well as a complete update on your deduction/co-payment status. If benefits are denied, you also have the right to know why, in writing.

Catastrophic coverage

If you can afford the premiums, it is a good idea to add a catastrophic policy to your health insurance umbrella—just in case. That's because some accidents or afflictions require a lifetime of medical care or rehabilitation services. For example, an auto accident can leave its victim paralyzed, requiring years of intensive rehabilitation. A stroke can render a person unable to speak, a condition that can sometimes be combated by cognitive and speech therapy.

Many policies don't cover these long-term, expensive treatments, which may be required if the patient is to have any hope of returning to a normal life. Thus, a catastrophic policy with a high lifetime benefit package can make a big difference in the life of a person who suffers such a tragedy.

Big Brother May Be Watching

A major plus of conventional health insurance policies has always been that they did not allow insurance company adjusters and executives to stick their corporate noses into what you and your doctor decided was best to promote your individual health needs. Well, thanks to either doctor greed or the insurance industry's "bottom line" mentality (depending on whom you talk to, doctors or insurance executives), you and your doctor now frequently have a back seat driver as you cruise down the health care highway of life—the medical review committee made up of physicians or nurses who review your records to determine if the tests or treatment you are planning on or receiving, are medically necessary.

Under this new way of doing business, many policies now require that you and your doctor obtain *prior or continuing approval* for many of the following:

- Nonemergency hospitalizations
- Nonemergency surgery, with second opinions often required
- Certain diagnostic tests, especially if given in a hospital
- The length of the hospitalization, once admitted. This means you could receive a written notice in your hospital bed that as of two days hence, all hospital bills are on you.
- The appropriateness of care given. This means that your doctor could be told after treating you that the procedures performed were not necessary and thus, will not be paid for. I am sure you can imagine the burden that can put on you.

Hint: Failure to comply with these restrictions can cause you to lose a portion or all of your benefits. So, while you are thinking about it, review your policy or call your agent or administrator to see what your pre-approval obligations are. Your future financial health may depend on it.

~ *The Blue Plate Special* ~

There is an old saying, "The times are changing and you've got to change with the times." As health care began to change under the banner of "cost effectiveness," a form of *prepaid* health care began to eat away at the near monopoly enjoyed by conventional health insurance providers. This "new concept" (it's really been around since the 1930s) is the Health Maintenance Organization, popularly known as the HMO.

HMOs provide their members with comprehensive health services for a fixed price which is paid in advance of receiving the covered medical care. Most large insurance carriers now offer some form of HMO to their customers and many very large companies or nonprofit organizations are in the HMO business almost exclusively.

Here's how the HMO concept works, at least in theory:

You pay the HMO (or your employer or union does in a group plan) a fixed sum, usually but not necessarily per month, after which you are known as a "plan member." The HMO is thereafter obligated to provide you with all of the medical services it has agreed to provide in your "plan," which generally includes primary care, specialty care, hospitalization and a broad range of other health services.

You are permitted only to use those physicians and facilities (hospitals, clinics, etc.) who are authorized to treat plan members for your non-emergency health care in order to qualify for HMO benefits.

In return, you pay nothing or at the most a nominal sum for these services regardless of the severity of your health problem. The key benefit for the plan member is nearly absolute health care cost control. No more deductibles and no more co-payments that can run into the thousands of dollars. In other words, one price pays for all of the rides.

Sound too good to be true? Well, some claim it is. These critics contend that HMOs make their money by withholding quality medical care through such tactics as delaying diagnostic tests, shortening hospital stays and refusing to authorize referrals from primary care physicians to more expensive sub-specialists.

The supporters of HMOs retort that the only things HMOs don't "give" to members are unnecessary testing and treatment, a policy that does not reduce the quality of care, just the expense. Plus, these defenders point out, there is far less paperwork to be processed in HMOs, since insurance forms don't have to be filled out. This reduction in paperwork, it is claimed, lowers the price the patient is paying the doctor or hospital for administrative costs, a price that is built in to each fee-for-service bill.

With all of the flak flying back and forth about HMOs, it is incumbent upon health care consumers who may be attracted to the concept to learn as much as they can about the HMOs that operate in their locality. The following information should provide a good starting point.

Variations On A Theme

Since nothing in life seems to be simple anymore, I'm sure that you have guessed that there is more than one "type" of HMO.

The Group Model: This type of HMO generally is a coming together of a large partnership of doctors called a "group" which contracts with a Health Plan to form the HMO. Sometimes, as with the Kaiser Permanente HMO in California, hospitals are also made a part of this partnership. Under this system, the plan refers exclusively to the medical group and the group treats only patients who are members of the plan. With rare exceptions, referrals to sub-specialists will be within the group. Decision-making is made jointly by the plan, the doctors, and when appropriate, the hospitals. Members usually must obtain their health care at plan hospitals or clinics.

The Staff Model: This type of HMO is owned by the health plan which employs the physicians. Physicians may have less clout with plan management concerning issues of quality of care since they are employed "one-on-one" rather than being partners with the plan as members of a large group of physicians. (Of course, those plans that pay no attention to issues of quality of care would have a hard time staying in business.) Like the group model, members of a staff model HMO usually must have all of their health needs attended to at plan clinics or hospitals, and the doctors work exclusively for the plan. Also, again with rare exceptions, all referrals to sub-specialists must be to other physician employees of the plan.

The IPA Model: IPA stands for "Independent Physician Association." An Independent Physician Association is an association of physicians in private practice that, for the limited purpose of working within an HMO setting, forms a legal entity which contracts with the Health Plan to provide services for plan members. Unlike group and staff models,

IPA physicians continue in private practice and treat HMO and non-HMO patients alike. That means that plan members visit private medical offices rather than hospitals or clinics for their normal medical care. The HMO also contracts with local hospitals to handle their plan members who need hospitalization. Patients of the HMO must receive their treatment from plan authorized doctors, their nonemergency hospitalization must be at contract hospitals, and all referrals to sub-specialists must be from within the IPA or as authorized by the plan.

HMOs vs. Conventional Policies

There really are significant differences between conventional health insurance plans and HMOs. Let's take a look.

On The One Hand

1. In HMOs, your *choice of physicians is limited* to those who are authorized by the plan, although that number can be significant. Under conventional fee-for-service policies, you can choose any doctor you want.

2. With HMOs, your *choice of sub-specialists will be restricted, and usually must be approved,* by the plan beforehand. With conventional policies, you are free to choose any sub-specialist you want, and will usually not have to get prior approval for the referral (although you may for the treatment).

3. With HMOs, *the sub-specialist is usually selected by the plan,* while with traditional fee-for-service policies, you choose.

4. Except in emergency situations (life-threatening) *you must use HMO hospitals* for all of your hospitalization needs. Under conventional health insurance plans, any hospital may be used although there may be reduced benefits in some hospitals if your company has hospitals under contract for use by its beneficiaries.

5. Unlike fee-for-service doctors, *your HMO primary care physician will generally not be available to you twenty-four hours a day* in staff or group models, although a physician who has access to your records will be.

6. *"Healthy care" services at HMOs are sometimes performed by nurse practitioners* or, in the case of obstetric care, certified nurse midwives. Obviously in fee-for-service plans you choose whether to have this alternate type of care.

7. If you go to a non-HMO facility *in an urgent care situation* (a medical condition requiring care within a day) *the facility will have to obtain prior approval from your HMO* before conducting tests or undertaking treatment if it expects to be paid. And unless things are serious, there's a good chance that your HMO will tell it to send you to an HMO facility, thus delaying your treatment. Under fee-for-service plans, you will usually be able to obtain the treatment seen as necessary by the emergency room medical team *immediately,* regardless of the hospital you go to.

8. *The same prior approval rules apply if you need medical treatment while outside your HMO's service area* (there are as yet no truly national HMOs). Under traditional health insurance there is no such thing as a "service area."

9. *If you have a doctor who is not an HMO physician, you will have to sever that relationship when you sign up.* Obviously, this doesn't happen with conventional policies.

Hint: If you are thinking of joining an IPA model HMO and already have a doctor whom you really like, ask if he or she is a member of any HMOs. If so, you can keep your costs contained without having to change doctors.

10. *Some members complain that their health care is short-changed* due to the pressure to keep costs down.

On The Other Hand

1. *You pay little or nothing for your treatment* in an HMO setting so long as you are a member in good standing.

2. *Most HMO plans include the price of medications.* Many fee-for-service insurance policies do not. And as you all probably know, most prescription medicines cost money, with a capital "M."

3. *HMOs not only allow preventive medicine and regular physicals, they encourage them.* Most conventional health policies *do not* pay for such treatment, thus discouraging their policy holders from attending to this important aspect of health care. (HMOs believe that the best way to keep costs down is to keep their members healthy, or at least, catch problems earlier rather than later — thus the term "Health Maintenance.")

4. While you can't choose any doctor to be your primary care physician, *the available pool of board-certified and board-qualified PCPs who may treat HMO members is usually quite large.* And most permit you to select your own doctor from within that pool.

5. *Sub-specialists to whom HMO members are referred to will generally have a good working rapport with the primary care physician,* while under fee-for-service plans, the sub-specialist you choose may not know your PCP.

6. *There is no personal financial disincentive for your doctor in an HMO to refer you to a sub-specialist or for a second opinion* since he or she will probably get paid the same amount regardless of the referral. Under fee-for-service plans, some doctors may prefer to hold on to the case for monetary reasons.

7. *In a group model HMO, there is a substantial amount of informal peer review since more than one doctor* within the group may treat you at different times. Also, the hard decisions are usually made in committee, and as they say, two (or three or four) heads are better than one.

8. So long as you seek treatment from HMO doctors and HMO hospitals, you don't have to worry about "Big Brother" telling you later that he won't pay. *Any unnecessary treatment you receive will be the responsibility of the HMO and the medical facility to thrash out.*

9. You can be sure that *you will not be subjected to unnecessary testing or medical procedures* as can be the case in fee-for-service care.

10. In group or staff models, *you have the convenience of "one-stop shopping,"* as all of your physicians and testing facilities will probably be located in one place. This also means your records are immediately available to all of your physicians, which allows for coordination of care.

11. *Most HMOs work on maintaining quality controls* since poor quality medical care will lead to loss of business. In the world of fee-for-service insurance, your insurance company has no control over quality of care, except perhaps in those situations where hospitals are under contract.

When asked to summarize the difference between HMOs and fee-for-service policies, an executive of one company used an analogy that I find very appropriate. He said that different people choose different health policies for different reasons, just as people choose different gas stations for different reasons. Some prefer the "full service" (traditional health insurance) island, and pay forty cents more per gallon for the extra service. Others prefer "self service" (HMOs and their progeny), getting the same gasoline and pocketing the difference. Neither is right nor wrong. It's all a matter of preference and an ability to pay.

Hint: The HMO industry is a growth industry, and thus there are a lot of different plans entering the marketplace. Unfortunately, not all of them are making it financially. Thus, when selecting an HMO (or any health insurance for that matter) make sure the plan is large enough and financially secure enough to stay in business over a long period of time. Otherwise you may pay the burden in premiums without receiving the benefit of prepaid health care.

(A good rule of thumb when looking for a financially stable HMO is to select one that has been in business for a long time and/or one that is backed by a large insurance company, although in a free enterprise system there are never any guarantees.)

Let's Go HMO Shopping

If you've decided that you are seriously interested in the HMO concept, here are some tips to help you find the best plan for you. What you are looking for is *quality*—quality of *care*, quality of *service* and quality of *coverage*.

Quality of care concerns the level of medical treatment you receive at the hands of HMO medical personnel and in HMO clinical facilities. You will want to ask the salesperson or plan administrator the following questions:

1. What credentials must a doctor possess to be on the HMO staff? You want an HMO that insists on board-qualified or board-certified physicians in each area of care.

2. Which hospitals does the HMO use? As a smart health care consumer, you should learn about the reputations of the hospitals in your area anyway. And if the HMO owns its own hospitals, try to find out their reputation. (For details on how to do this, see Chapter 8.) If your HMO contracts with local hospitals, it will obviously make a difference if the contract hospitals have nicknames like "St. Gangrene" or "Staph Infection Medical Center."

3. How many doctors are available for me to choose from? Obviously, the bigger the pool the better your chance of selecting the physician who is right for you.

4. Can I choose my own PCP, and if not, how easy is it to change doctors? Obviously, if you get stuck with a doctor you don't trust or whom you can't stand, you will not use that doctor, thereby destroying one of the prime benefits of HMO care, the availability of low-cost preventive medicine. Most HMOs allow you to change doctors freely, but ask just in case.

5. Can I see the same doctor every time? The whole point of having a primary care physician is to have personalized care available when you need it. Of course, in staff and group model HMOs, if you have unexpected health problems that require immediate attention, your PCP may not be available.

6. How many sub-specialists are available, should I need one? Ready access to good sub-specialists is important. Thus if the HMO only has one heart surgeon or one gastroenterologist whom it permits its members to use, you may wish to look around for a different HMO.

7. Is home nursing care available if I need it? Since the emphasis in HMOs is admittedly on cost-cutting, you may find that you are given ambulatory treatment when a fee-for-service patient might get a day or two of hospitalization. And so home nursing care should be available to you without charge.

8. What is the grievance procedure? In an HMO there may come a time when you feel you are not getting the quality of care you deserve. Perhaps you feel that certain diagnostic tests should be performed and the HMO disagrees. Or, perhaps you believe you should be hospitalized while the HMO determines that your ailment can be adequately treated on an outpatient basis. You will want a grievance procedure that you can understand and readily use to appeal that decision.

Hint: If such disputes take place, you can usually receive the care you want and then squabble later over who pays. So, if you feel strongly about an issue of quality care, go for quality and worry about money later. After all, unlike cats, we humans live but once.

---

9. What is the HMO policy with regard to emergency care? In an emergency situation, you want an HMO which has a policy of protecting your health first and worrying about the bottom line later. Make sure that if you must go to a non-HMO emergency room on an emergency or urgent care basis that HMO red tape won't foul up your treatment.

Quality of service deals with matters of convenience and courtesy. Before you sign up, call one of the HMO hospitals and see if it is possible to get through to the department you want without having to wait forever. See if the phones are answered in a courteous way and whether you are treated with respect. Ask to take a tour of one of the hospitals (especially in a staff or group model) to see if it is efficiently run or if it looks like a stockyard with all of the patients milling around waiting to be helped. You might also want to ask some of the following questions.

1. How many HMO hospitals are available near my home and work? This is especially important in emergency and urgent care matters. After all, you don't want to have to drive for forty-five minutes to get to an HMO facility while feeling nauseous.

2. How long is the usual wait before seeing the doctor? Some HMOs have the reputation of moving the work along about as fast as the Long Island Expressway moves at rush hour. Thus, in a non-IPA situation, it might be a good idea to tour the facility you will be using to see exactly what you are getting yourself into.

3. Where is the doctor's office that I will be using? Some HMOs have clinics that are for outpatient services which may be in a different location than the hospital. The accessibility to the clinic will be important, as will its proximity to bus lines if you must use public transportation. If you join an IPA model, you will want to make sure that private practitioners affiliated with the HMO practice are near enough to you to keep you from having to drive all over town in search of medical care.

Quality of coverage is what makes an HMO worthwhile. An HMO that has a broad range of services available to you for the one price means that you truly *do* control your health care expenses. On the other hand, an HMO with limited service benefits defeats the whole purpose.

The best way to evaluate competing HMOs regarding quality of coverage is to ask each for a "spread sheet" and compare the service offered in each with the price of the policy. Here's an example:

Benefits	**HMO #1 ($226 Mo.)**	**HMO #2 ($210 Mo.)**	**HMO #3 ($163 Mo.)**
Office Visits	Free	Free	$10
Surgery	Free	Free	Free
Maternity Care	Free	Free	$8.00 Per Visit
Alcohol/Drug Dependency	Free	$50	Unavailable
Home Health Services	Free	$5	Unavailable
Immunizations	Free	Free	Free
Vision Exams	Free	Free	$10
Diagnostic Tests In Hospital	Free	Free	Free

Ambulance	Free	Free	Free
Lab Tests	Free	Free	Free
Hospitalization	Free	Free	80% of costs first 5 days, then, free.

By comparing the services you receive with the price you pay, you will be able to find the HMO that best matches your budget and provides the services you need.

Hint: Most of us receive our health insurance through our employment or union affiliation. Usually, there will be more than one plan offered to you, be it HMOs, conventional health insurance or some other form of protection. Always ask for spread sheets before selecting to better enable yourself to choose the right plan to suit your needs.

Hint: Many HMOs sell a large number of memberships to plan brokers at reduced group prices. If you are not a member of a group, you still may be able to find discount prices by utilizing the services of such a broker, who will sell the plan at a profit but still under the individual policy price.

Hint: As with all health insurance, make sure the HMO can't cancel your membership because of reasons of health.

~ *À La Carte* ~

IPAs: Independent Practice Associations are not limited to working with HMOs. Many times, these organizations contract on their own with local hospitals to provide fixed rate care and then market their own health plans to employee groups or the public in what might be termed a mini-HMO.

PPOs: Preferred Provider Organizations are a hybrid form of conventional health insurance in which a group insurance carrier contracts with hospitals and doctor group practices to steer its policyholders to the members of the PPO, in return for which they give discount fees for medical care. The plan is not a prepaid medical service like an HMO or an IPA, but is a traditional fee-for-service plan where the trade-off for lowered prices is a limitation on the choice of physicians and medical facilities. If a patient whose coverage is in the form of a PPO goes to a non-PPO doctor or facility, he or she must pay the difference between what the insurance company would have paid a PPO doctor and what the treating physician actually charges. Most PPO doctors must accept what the insurance company pays as payment in full from the patient, although in some plans there will be a deductible and/or co-payment obligation.

Most PPOs operate under the "Big Brother school" of health cost-containment, and thus require pre-approval in many medical situations such as nonemergency admissions to hospitals. That means if a dispute arises over the appropriateness of certain treatment, you may end up holding the bill.

Medicare and Medicaid: Yes, the government does have a health care heart (although of shrinking proportions in recent years) that it expresses through the Medicare and Medicaid programs of health care financing.

Medicare

Medicare is a federal health insurance plan that provides basic protection for those entitled to receive benefits, currently, those sixty-five or older who have paid Social Security taxes and their eligible spouses, or those who receive Railroad Retirement benefits. In addition, persons who have been entitled to receiving Social Security disability benefits for at least two years and anyone who has permanent or chronic kidney failure requiring dialysis is also eligible for benefits.

The primary purpose of Medicare is to reduce the burden of the costs of medical care to Americans in their "golden years." Unfortunately, the system has in many ways become more iron pyrite than gold, since the elderly now, on average, pay more out of their pockets for medical care than they did before the inception of the program. But as the old saying goes, "any port in a storm," and with health care costs reaching virtual hurricane proportions, the program is still a very valuable one, indeed.

Medicare comes in two parts:

Part A is a compulsory form of hospital insurance that comes, at least for now, at no cost to its beneficiaries (being paid by Social Security taxes). During each "benefit period" (which begins when an insured person enters a hospital and ends when he or she has not been in a hospital or skilled nursing facility for 60 days), Part A will pay for the following:

1. Ninety days of inpatient care subject to a deductible which is currently over $500, and which is subject to change (almost certainly in the wrong direction for the patient). A daily co-payment is required from day sixty-one through day ninety in the amount of $130, and it is climbing. An additional lifetime reserve of sixty days is available, with the daily co-payment virtually doubling during that period.

2. Up to 100 days in a skilled nursing facility for persons in need of skilled nursing or rehabilitation services. This benefit also requires a daily co-payment, currently at sixty-five dollars. NOTE: This benefit is for skilled nursing care only. It does *not* provide for chronic long-term care such as is usually provided in those facilities we tactfully call "convalescent homes."

3. Home health services requiring skilled medical care are provided for a limited period of time without any co-payments being required (at least for now).

4. Hospice care for the terminally ill (who otherwise qualify) is available (also for a limited time) with the only co-payment requirements being for medication. If a Medicare recipient elects to follow this route for his or her illness, he or she must receive the services through a hospice and give up the other Medicare benefits.

Payments for hospitalization are now made on the basis of DRGs (diagnosis related groups). This system provides for payments to be made to hospitals at a predetermined specified rate, which represents the average cost nationwide of treating other patients with the same diagnosis. This means that a hospital financially benefits the *sooner* a Medicare patient is released, rather than later.

Defenders of the DRG system claim that the discharge date from a hospital is to be made on the basis of the Medicare recipient's medical needs alone and not on the amount the hospital receives by way of DRG payment. Unfortunately, Medicare recipients have to live in the real world, and according to many of the doctors I have talked to, in the real world the DRG system is, at least occasionally, misused, leading to insufficient medical care. Therefore, if you believe that you or a loved one who is receiving Medicare benefits are being discharged before it is medically appropriate to do so, remember the following:

1. You *do,* under the law, have the right to receive all of the hospital care necessary for the proper diagnosis and treatment of the illness or injury, regardless of whether the hospital makes a profit off of your care.

2. You have the right to be fully informed about decisions affecting your Medicare coverage and your medical treatment. Get these decisions in writing whenever possible and get copies of the medical records if you believe a dispute concerning hospitalization is likely to occur.

3. You have the right to *appeal* written notices you receive from the hospital or Medicare stating that your hospitalization will no longer be covered. *Unless the notice is in writing, there is no right to appeal, so never accept an oral representation!* Be sure that the written notice details how an appeal is to be processed. That is your right under the law.

4. If you decide to appeal, don't delay. You will be dealing with what is called a Peer Review Organization (PRO) which has the responsibility of reviewing the appropriateness and quality of hospital treatment. Call your local PRO immediately and don't leave the hospital if you and your doctor believe that such a move will jeopardize your health. If your appeal is victorious, you will continue to receive benefits for care; if not, the bill for the extra days of hospitalization will soon arrive in the mail.

Part B is a voluntary program of supplemental medical insurance coverage, somewhat equivalent to a Major Medical health insurance policy in that it partially covers the cost of services such as surgery, office visits, diagnostic testing and the use of durable medical equipment. Medicare recipients must pay a small monthly fee in order to be covered, either through direct payments or deductions from their Social Security checks.

Payments to physicians under Part B are based on what is called a "reasonable" charge, an amount which is invariably less than the actual charge made by the doctor for the services rendered. Medicare will pay eighty percent of the reasonable charge after the Medicare beneficiary has paid a deductible, which is currently under $100. If the physician agrees to "accept" the Medicare assignment, he or she will be paid directly by Medicare, under the stipulation that the reasonable charge will be deemed the full charge to the patient for the service. If the doctor does *not* accept the assignment, the Medicare benefit is paid directly to the patient, who is responsible to pay the doctor's actual charge. In both cases, the Medicare payment (whether to patient or doctor) will be eighty percent of the reasonable charge. Here's how all of the mumbo-jumbo works in the real world:

	M.D. Accepts Assignment	**M.D. Does Not Accept Assignment**
M.D.'s Charge	$1,000	$1,000
"Reasonable" Charge Allowed by Medicare	$750	$750
Medicare Pays M.D.	$600 (80% of $750)	n/a
Medicare Pays Patient	n/a	$600*
Net Cost to Patient	$150 ($750 minus $600)	$400** ($1,000 minus $600)

*minus deductible if not already paid
**plus deductible if not already paid

Hint: Not all doctors accept Medicare patients and many of those who do will not accept the Medicare payment as payment in full. So if you are a Medicare beneficiary on a limited budget, you may find that your choice of doctors is somewhat limited. So, the magic question to ask the doctor becomes, "*Do you accept Medicare payments as payment in full?*"

Hint: Medicare does not pay for routine care. Thus, if your doctor does not come up with a diagnosis, you are on your own.

Medigap Insurance: Medigap policies are intended to pay for that portion of medical treatment to Medicare beneficiaries that the program itself does not pay for. (You can always tell a Medigap policy advertisement—it will be the one featuring a former big-time actor whose hair has turned gray.) As with any insurance program, read the fine print *before* you sign up, especially with regard to pre-existing conditions, renewal and exclusions.

Hint: If you qualify for Medicaid protection in your state because of low income, you may be able to avoid having to purchase a supplemental policy.

Hint: Look for policies that do not limit their benefits to the "reasonable" fee permitted by Medicare. In other words, you want a policy that pays benefits based on the doctor's *actual charge.* The difference in the two is a distinction with a definite difference, a difference of up to forty percent of the fee.

HMOs and Medicare: Many HMOs now offer their plans to Medicare recipients. If you sign up as a plan member, Medicare pays the HMO a monthly fee for your care and you may have to pay a small fee to cover the deductible and co-payment obligation. In return, you become an HMO plan member, with all of the benefits and restrictions that entails. In return, you *give up* your other Medicare benefits. In other words, you must use HMO facilities and otherwise comply with the plan rules. (According to many of the health care professionals I talked to, many Medicare HMO plan members don't understand that they can no longer go to *any* doctor or hospital, so if you or a loved one has opted for this course of health care protection, be sure you understand the rules.)

A Final Note About Medicare:

The rules under which the program is operated undergo constant change. Even as I write this, Congress is actively debating about reducing the out-of-pocket expenses that recipients will have to pay and extending the coverage maximums so as to provide comprehensive medical care. There is also talk of extending Medicare to cover nursing home care, which it does not do at present. And so, since the law can change far quicker than this book can be revised, be sure to ask your local Social Security Office about the specific Medicare benefits and deductibles which may apply to you.

Medicaid

Medicaid is a federally aided, state-operated and administered program of health care assistance for the poor who are aged, blind, disabled or members of families with dependent children. All states except Arizona participate in Medicaid (although Arizona has an alternative program). The name of each program varies from state to state.

Because the programs rely on partial state funding and upon state administration, the range of services vary greatly from locality to locality, but it is pretty safe to say that eligible persons must be either receiving welfare or Social Security SSI (Supplemental Security Income) benefits or must be entitled to receive them. Pregnant women who will qualify for assistance once their child is born also qualify for benefits regarding the pregnancy.

The following programs will, at minimum, be offered to qualified Medicaid recipients:

- Inpatient and outpatient hospital services
- Lab and x-ray services
- Skilled nursing care, at home if necessary
- Family Planning services, and
- Physicians' services

Medicaid recipients may also be entitled to prescription drug benefits, eyeglasses and intermediate care facilities.

Hint: Not all physicians or medical facilities are willing to treat Medicaid beneficiaries. To find who will in your locality, contact your state or local Health Department, which will also be able to tell you if you qualify for benefits in your state.

Miscellaneous

There are other methods by which health care is financed in the United States today. Here is a list of some of the more notable:

Veterans Hospitals: Some, but certainly not all, veterans of the armed forces have the right to "socialized medicine" through Veterans Administration hospitals and clinics (and on rare occasions through private physicians). You are probably eligible if you:

- Have "service-connected" medical or dental conditions
- Have a service-related disability
- Are eligible for Medicaid
- Are in receipt of a Veterans Administration pension
- Are a former POW or are a Vietnam veteran who needs treatment for a condition possibly related to exposure to dioxin or other toxic substances such as Agent Orange
- Are an "Atomic Veteran," (those exposed to radiation during atomic tests or during the occupation of Hiroshima or Nagasaki), for treatment of conditions possibly related to exposure to radiation.

Low-income veterans and their dependents may be provided hospital treatment for non-service-related medical conditions on a space available basis, or, if ineligible for free care, may receive services upon the condition that they pay a co-payment.

Remember, like Medicare, the rules of VA care are subject to change. Thus be sure to consult your local Veterans Administration Office if you have any questions about eligibility or services.

Free/Community Clinics: Most large cities and some rural communities have free clinics that provide free medical care to anyone who walks through the door. There are also community clinics that will charge on a sliding scale based on ability to pay. Convenient care may not be available in these facilities, but quality care usually is, so don't allow yourself to go untreated because you have no money to pay.

NOTE: These clinics generally do not provide emergency or long-term care, their main emphasis being on preventive medicine and general care.

Foundations: Many charitable foundations, such as The Muscular Dystrophy Association, provide medical and financial benefits for persons who suffer from specific afflictions. If you or someone you love has been diagnosed with having such a disease, ask your doctor if there are such services available to you.

General Hospitals: Everyone is entitled to receive treatment at public medical facilities which go under the generic name, general hospital. Admission will usually be through the emergency room. The quality of care varies from hospital to hospital, some being the medical equivalent of The Promised Land while others make the Black Hole of Calcutta seem like a country club.

Stand Up For Your Rights

Now I know that insurance companies are bigger than you are, that they own high-rise office buildings and that they each have enough lawyers on retainer to choke a whale. But that does not mean you can't play David to their Goliath. All you have to do is be willing to "grab your sling" and assert yourself.

If you believe that your health insurance company has denied you benefits to which you are entitled under the terms of your policy, take action.

If the company denies a claim, it will be in writing and it will tell you the review procedures you can take within the company to "appeal" the denial. Follow those procedures and assert your rights presenting as much "objective" evidence as possible, such as medical records and copies of claim forms. Ask your doctor to help you with your records or by writing a report.

If you cannot get satisfaction and you feel strongly enough about the matter to play hardball—hire a lawyer. Among the actions your lawyer may wish to take (if you have a case) are:

• *Writing a Letter*–Sometimes a letter from a lawyer can accomplish things that a letter from a non-lawyer cannot. The cost will be relatively inexpensive and the matter may be solved then and there.

• *Suing for Breach of Contract*–Your insurance policy is a contract, and if your company breaches it, you can sue for damages which will probably, but not necessarily, be your out-of-pocket monetary losses. Most insurance policies also provide for the payment of attorney fees in the event of breach, which means that if you win, the company may also be ordered to pay for all or part of your lawyer's fees. Of course you may lose, so be sure you have a good case before taking this step.

• *Suing for "Bad Faith"*–Bad Faith litigation is a relatively recent development in the law that permits "wronged" insurance policy holders to sue for damages far in excess of what they suffered "out of pocket." The idea here is that insurance companies should be punished by assessing "punitive damages" against them if they treat their beneficiaries in "bad faith," that is, in an arbitrary, malicious or vindictive manner, such as denying a valid claim without conducting a good faith investigation. (Believe me, it happens.) Bad Faith will not apply if your insurance company has acted reasonably in handling your claim (meaning in good faith), but if you believe that you have been cheated with "malice aforethought," you can sue for big bucks, especially if your health or emotional state has been materially effected. (Thanks to a recent U.S. Supreme Court decision, you may not be able to sue your health insurance carrier for bad faith if you receive the health insurance as a benefit of employment.)

Hint: Whenever you deal with insurance companies, do so in writing and keep copies of all letters, claims and especially policies. In another forum, those documents will be called "evidence."

Hint: Many claims are validly denied and cause "hard feelings" only because the purchaser has not read or understood the policy. Thus, it is very important that you understand what you are buying—and not buying—ahead of time. After all, the worst time to find out that the safety net you thought was protecting you is really full of holes, is when you are counting on it to catch you.

NOTES TO THE CHART

Having had experience with HMOs, PPOs and IPAs during my professional career, I am a strong believer in fee-for-service medicine and traditional health insurance. This is because fee-for-service medicine gives the patient *choices,* which is to say the patient can choose any physician he or she wants, any sub-specialist and frequently, any hospital. Doctors can be changed at will without hassles and having to explain the reason to some plan administrator. In other words, you the patient have the best opportunity to find the best doctor for you. Granted, fee-for-service medicine is generally more expensive than HMO care or other health insurance programs.

I know of what I speak. After my residency, I worked for an HMO and I vividly recall the frustration I had to go through to get "permission" to hospitalize a patient that I believed was in acute need of hospitalization. I continue to hear rumors about these "battles royal" today.

IPA and PPO plans lie between fee-for-service and HMO practice. While there are financial advantages to these plans for patients, there is still a limitation on choice. But, as the old saying goes, "you get what you pay for."

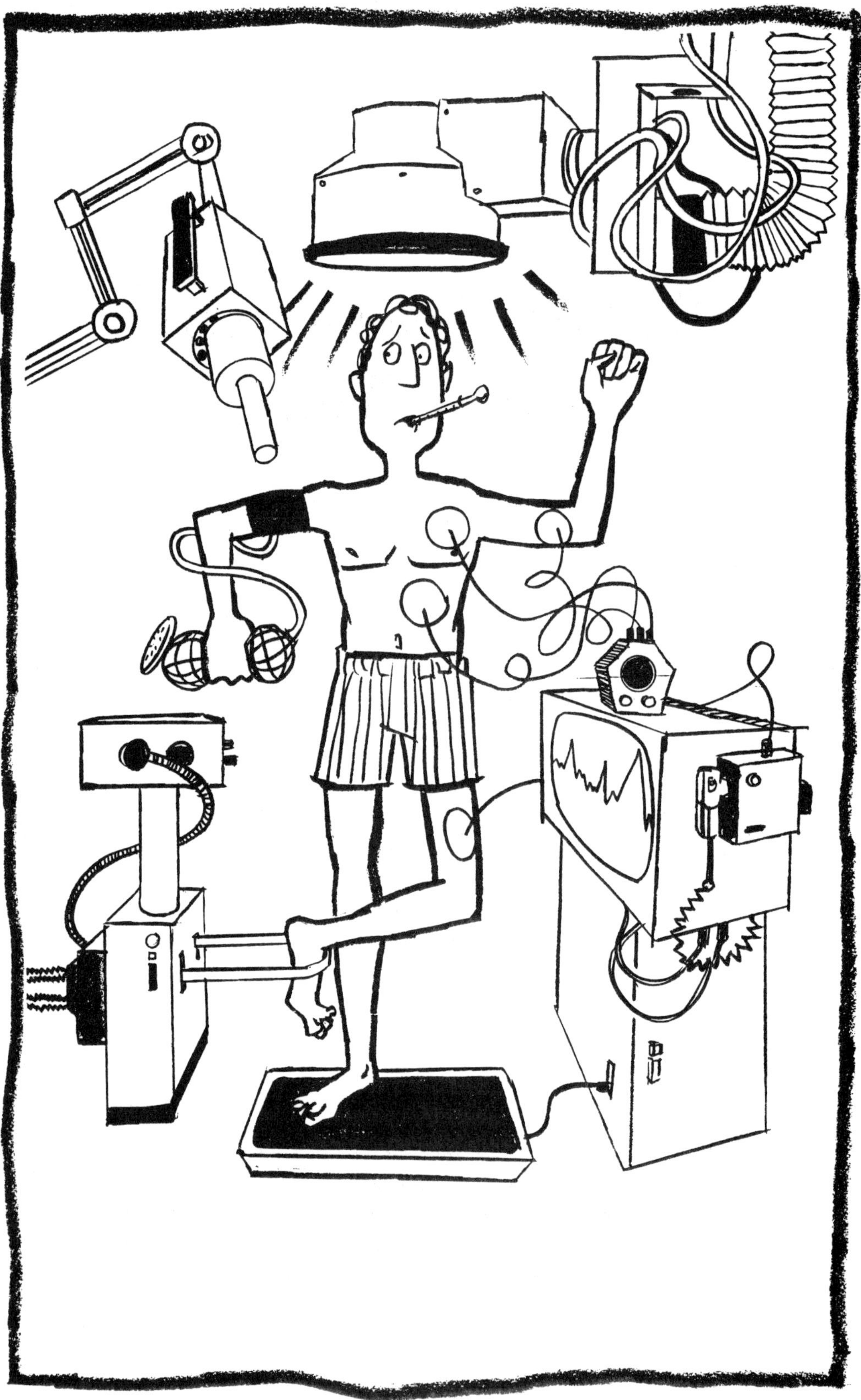

·6·

CHAPTER

Tests, Tests And More Tests

• The Physical Exam •

Our bodies are very complicated and wondrous organisms that make the intricate workings of a Swiss watch look like a child's wind-up toy. And like most complicated machinery, we need regular inspections and maintenance in order to keep the mechanism running smoothly. Doctors call this schedule of maintenance and repair "preventive medicine."

The "mechanic" who works hand-in-hand with you to prevent major breakdowns before they occur is usually your primary care physician. Part of his or her job is to establish a plan of preventive care specifically designed to take into account your health, your health history and any other factors, such as smoking, which your doctor believes to be of significance.

• The Normal Check Up •

The heart of any preventive medicine program is a consistent program of undergoing normal "routine" checkups. I use the term "routine" because it refers to healthy asymptomatic exams which are designed to ensure that you are actually in as good a shape as you may feel. The healthy physical examination normally consists of the following parts:

History

The health history of a patient is one of the most important factors doctors use in analyzing the potential health problems that may face their patients. And so, during your examination with a physician, you will probably be asked to supply some of the following information:

Family History: When deciding upon a course of preventive medicine, one of the things a doctor needs to do is identify any potential "weak links" in his or her patient's "chain" of health. Since the propensity to suffer certain medical difficulties may be genetic (as in some forms of heart disease or cancer), it is important for your doctor to know about the health history of your immediate family. For example, if there is a high incidence of polyps (a polite word for tumors) of the colon in your family, your doctor needs to be alerted to that fact so that he or she will know to keep a closer watch on your colon than would otherwise be the case. The same thing holds true of cancer, heart disease and, of course, proven hereditary diseases such as sickle-cell anemia. If you *don't* know the details of your parents', grandparents', aunts', uncles' or cousins' health histories, do some research. You may not win a Pulitzer Prize for your efforts, but you may be rewarded with a longer and healthier life.

Personal History: As we've discussed in previous chapters, our lifestyles often dictate the future course of our health. This means that your doctor needs to know about who you are and how you live your life, and in intimate detail. Thus, he or she will probably ask "personal" questions such as if you smoke, drink or take drugs. Your "love life" or lack thereof is also likely to be discussed, as well as if you are single, married, widowed or divorced. Your dietary habits, sleep patterns, whether you are happy in your career or profession, can all be issues your doctor finds relevant to your individual health. In such matters, the order of the day is candor, so be prepared to discuss these issues in a frank and non-defensive manner. After all, your doctor isn't interested in these things for kicks, but for health—*your* health.

Your doctor will also want details of your medical past, such as:

- Whether you have ever been hospitalized, and if so, when, for what reason, what treatment was given and the outcome

- If you have had prior illnesses, the dates of such illnesses and the method and outcome of treatment. This includes the usual childhood illnesses such as chicken pox, which may be a "rite of passage" in children, but which can be very serious in adults.

- A complete list of allergies and symptoms created by those things you may be allergic to

• Medical procedures you may have undergone such as abortions, plastic surgery, blood transfusions or the removal of cysts

Knowledge of these and other matters can alert your doctor to keep an eye out for certain problems and can also assist him or her in making a quick and accurate diagnosis should you become ill or otherwise suffer from symptoms of poor health.

History of current symptoms: If you are getting a physical because you are not feeling well, be sure you are able to provide an in-depth history of your symptoms with as much attention to time and detail as possible. Remember, the more accurate and detailed the information you give your doctor, the better able he or she will be to provide you with the medical answers you are looking for.

Hint: When we are ill, we usually suppress the problem and make the best of the hand we have been dealt. As a result, we may forget to tell our doctor about every symptom we may have experienced. To make sure this doesn't happen to you, try keeping a diary and bring it with you to the doctor's. In that way, you will be able to give your doctor the complete story.

The Physical Examination

All of us have at one time or another undergone a routine physical examination. However, most of us don't really know what all of that poking, prodding and inserting may be all about. And so, here's a brief rundown of what happens and *why* during a physical examination:

Hint: *Don't rely on this or any other book to answer all of your questions about your health* or what your doctor may or should be doing. If you don't understand something and you want to know why—ASK. Remember, it doesn't show that you are stupid when you ask questions, it shows that you are *smart*!

1. Your temperature is taken. A person whose temperature runs higher or lower than his or her norm (remember 98.6 degrees may be the norm, but some of us as individuals have body temperatures which naturally run higher or lower), may indicate the possibility of an illness, infection or disease.

2. Your "general appearance" is noted. Health and ill-health have certain "looks" which your doctor comes to recognize through training and experience. This is especially true if you have a long-term relationship with a doctor, who will learn to know your "look" very well, which again underscores the importance of a personal primary care physician.

3. You are weighed. Our weight can tell a lot about our health prospects. Someone who is gaining an unhealthy amount of weight may not only be putting undue pressure on his or her body, but the weight gain itself may be an indication of other problems such as stress, alcoholism, a thyroid condition or diabetes. Likewise, unexplained loss of weight may indicate a serious physical malady such as cancer. In any event, with so many of us experiencing weight problems or eating disorders in this country, an important part of our doctor's job is to advise us on matters of diet, nutrition and weight management.

4. Your blood pressure is taken to make sure it is within your personal "normal" range. This simple, painless test should be taken by everyone on a routine periodic basis, as it is really the only way to detect the presence of "the silent killer," hypertension. Hypertension is called the silent killer because it generally has no symptoms. Yet, over time, high blood pressure can so abuse internal organs that they may fail, leading to severe disability or death. Some of the "target" organs or body parts of hypertension are the heart, brain, arteries and kidneys. And while it is certainly true that "you gotta have heart," it is also true that "you gotta have kidneys."

5. Your respiration and pulse rates are counted. The number of heart beats per minute and the number of times you breathe per minute give the doctor a general indication of the shape your cardiovascular system is in. In addition, heart rhythm problems can sometimes be discovered as well as other heart abnormalities from the "feel" of the pulse, which is simply the way your blood courses through your arteries as pushed by the beating of your heart.

> **Hint:** All of the foregoing tests are usually conducted by a nurse or other qualified medical professional on behalf of the doctor. Don't be angry if the doctor doesn't conduct these tests personally, since this allows the physician to work more efficiently. Also, don't be upset if your doctor repeats a test "just to be sure," which he or she may do, especially if your doctor is "following" a condition such as high blood pressure.

6. The Head and Face Exam:

Eyes—Your doctor looks into your eyes using a tiny beam of light from a tool called an ophthalmoscope. Among the purposes of this procedure is to check pupil reaction and the general condition of your eyes. Abnormalities which may be noted can tell a doctor far more than the general health of your eyes. For example, early signs of brain disease may be observable in the eyes as can diseases of some organs, such as the liver. Also, the general condition of your blood vessels may be indicated by the shape of your eye capillaries.

Your doctor may also ask you to follow his or her finger with your eyes. Difficulties coordinating this motor skill may be an indication of muscle disease, such as multiple sclerosis, or a "silent" stroke or brain tumor.

Ears—Your ears are examined to make sure your eardrum is not perforated and to ensure that your ear canals are not obstructed.

Nose—Generally, unless there are problems of the nose or nasal passages, your nose is left pretty much alone during a routine physical.

Mouth and Throat—Your doctor puts a tongue depressor in your mouth and asks you to say "aah." The doctor can then observe many serious conditions of the mouth that have minor or no symptoms at all. These include cancers of the mouth and tongue, which can be deadly if not caught at an early stage, and mouth infections which may be early indications of disease, including AIDS.

7. The Neck Exam: The body is such a complex machine that even a seemingly simple part like the neck has within it intricate body parts, which, if abnormal, can indicate the presence of a serious medical condition. Your doctor "palpates" (feels) your neck to see if any of your lymph nodes are swollen, which could be an early indicator of a viral infection or cancer, and he or she also probably checks out your thyroid gland, which is found just below the "Adam's apple," to make sure it is not enlarged. He or she also looks for distended veins, which may be an indication of heart disease.

8. The Upper Trunk Exam:
Underarms—Our underarms are more important than being mere receptacles for deodorant products—they house lymph glands, which, as in the neck, are part of the waste-disposing lymphatic system. Thus the doctor "feels" for swollen lymph nodes which may not hurt, but whose presence may indicate a serious problem.

Chest—Your heart is listened to by means of a stethoscope (usually cold) to detect problems ranging from rhythm abnormalities to heart valve disease (a heart murmur). Your doctor also looks at your chest to see if there are any skeletal abnormalities and feels for your heart "PMI" (point of maximum impulse). If it is in the wrong place, this may indicate an enlarged heart. The "sound" your chest cavity makes when your doctor taps it can tell your doctor if things are copacetic, or whether further investigations into the heart, lungs or other organs should be made.

Breasts—A woman's breasts (and sometimes the breasts of a man) are palpitated in a methodical way so as to rub the tissues of the breast against the chest wall, to see whether there are any "marbles" (lumps) or growths present which could indicate the presence of breast cancer. This procedure is generally done with you in two positions: sitting up and lying down.

Back—Your doctor listens to your lungs with the still-cold stethoscope and listens to the percussion (sounds) your back makes when methodically tapped at key spots. Any abnormalities such as a wheezing of the lungs will alert the doctor to take a closer look. Your doctor also inspects the spine and palpates the muscles of the back.

9. The Abdominal Exam: Your doctor asks you to lie back on the examining table so that he or she can closely inspect the soft tissues of the abdomen. The doctor will deeply palpate to feel if any of the internal organs are enlarged or if the touch causes you pain. He or she will also look to see if there are any distensions or bulges which could indicate internal problems, and will probably listen to the bowel with the now warmer stethoscope to make sure the sounds of digestion are normal.

10. Genital Exam: Women will receive a pelvic exam which will consist of many parts. (Note: Women should be draped and a nurse should be present during a pelvic examination. Disposable gloves should be worn by the doctor at all times. If your doctor doesn't follow these procedures, demand that they be complied with before submitting to the examination.)

The external genitalia will be observed to see if there are any growths or sores which could indicate infection or veneral disease, then a woman's internal organs will be felt and/or looked at (with the assistance of an instrument called a speculum which separates the vaginal walls) to see whether there are any abnormal discharges, growths, discoloration of tissues or sores in the vagina, cervix or uterus, which may indicate anything from an infection to cysts or tumors, benign or malignant (cancerous). The doctor will also engage in a "bimanual" internal exam of the ovaries and uterus by feeling the abdomen with one hand while having two gloved fingers inserted into the vagina with the other. He or she may also conduct a rectovaginal exam to better examine the tone and alignment of the pelvic organs and to feel for abnormal growths. A pap test will also be conducted by scraping the cervix; the tissue is then evaluated by a pathologist or lab to see whether there are any abnormal cells, which could be a warning sign of cancer.

Hint: You have a right to know what the doctor is doing and *why*, every step of the way. So when in doubt, ask your doctor to go slowly and explain the purpose behind every aspect of the pelvic examination before it is conducted. Also, if you feel your doctor is being unduly rough or if he or she is hurting you, say so. You have the absolute right to be treated gently and with respect.

Hint: If you feel uncomfortable about anything your doctor may be doing during a pelvic examination, ask questions rather than suffer in silence. If you don't like the answer or if you feel you have been abused, contact another expert in the field or a feminist health clinic to see whether your examination was conducted properly.

Men have their genitals inspected for abnormal growths, swelling or sores which could indicate the presence of a tumor or veneral disease. The doctor also places his or her fingers underneath the scrotum and asks the patient to cough to check for the presence of a hernia.

11. The Rectal Exam: Your doctor inserts a gloved finger into the rectum to check for growth or blood which could be a sign of a malignancy in the rectum or colon. Men will also have their prostate gland massaged to check for enlargement or growths.

12. Miscellaneous: Your doctor looks at your legs, arms, hands and feet to check for swelling or other signs of problems. Reflex tests may also be taken (after which you may feel like wrapping that rubber hammer around your doctor's throat). And your skin is examined for growths, discolorations or changes in moles.

Preventive Screening

The physical exam usually takes between thirty and forty-five minutes, and should do a pretty thorough job of checking out your machinery. However, the physical exam in and of itself may fall short of catching illness and disease earlier rather than later. For a truly complete job, your doctor should also take or order some screening tests, which provide an even closer look at your system and the way it is operating.

Here are some of the typical tests which your doctor may wish to have performed:

Stool Slide Test: This is an analysis of the stool in search of hidden traces of blood, the appearance of which can be an early sign of cancer somewhere in the digestive tract.

Sigmoidoscopies: These procedures go the digital rectal exam one better by permitting the physician to actually see inside the colon by means of a flexible tube which is inserted into the colon. While the test is certainly not fun, it can prove invaluable at catching cancer at a very early stage, thereby vastly increasing the odds of a complete cure.

Mammogram: In essence, a mammogram is an x-ray of the breast which searches for lumps that may be too small to locate manually. The key target is cancer, again on the sound theory that the earlier the detection, the more likely the cure.

Hint: The American Cancer Society recommends that women above the age of twenty conduct breast self-examinations once a month. Obviously, if a lump is detected, don't wait in hopes that it will go away, but immediately contact your doctor. For details of the proper method of self-examination, ask your primary care physician, ob/gyn, your local women's health center or your local chapter of The American Cancer Society.

Pap Test: As described earlier, the Pap test seeks to catch cancer of the uterus or cervix at the earliest possible moment.

Chest x-ray: X-rays of the chest seek to uncover problems of the lungs such as TB, tumors and diseases caused by industrial pollution.

Hint: If you are or even think you may be pregnant, be sure to tell the x-ray technician so that a protective cover can be placed over your reproductive organs—or choose not to have the x-ray at all.

EKG: Short for electrocardiogram, an EKG charts the beating and rhythm of the heart so that the doctor can see whether there are any irregularities or changes from previous EKGs.

Cardiac Stress Test: Popularly known as a "treadmill," this procedure examines how well the heart works when it is forced to beat fast in response to exercise (stress).

Blood Test: Your blood can tell a physician many things about how the organs of the body are doing their jobs and can signal dysfunctions (breakdowns) before they have displayed any symptoms. Here are just a few of the tests that can be run on blood.

1. A blood count measures the quantity of red blood cells to white blood cells and measures the presence of the differing types of white blood cells. An abnormal ratio of white to red may alert your doctor to problems that may soon appear on the horizon. For example, an excess of white blood cells may mean that your body is trying to fight off an infection.

2. A thyroid function test will catch potential problems of the thyroid before any symptoms appear.

3. The "biochemical profile" tells your doctor many things about many different parts of the body, including cholesterol levels—important for preventing heart disease—and the levels of other blood substances which can indicate malfunctions of the liver and kidneys, just to name a few.

4. The exposure to syphilis, AIDS, and other venereal diseases can be detected by testing the blood.

Hint: Just because you receive a blood test does not mean that every test will be undertaken with the sample given. Ask your doctor which tests will be conducted and the purpose for each, if you have any questions.

Urinalysis: Like blood, urine is a veritable window to the workings of the vital organs, particularly the kidneys and the entire urinary tract.

If your screening tests all prove to be negative and your physical examination shows no problems, the chances are good (but not 100 percent) that you are in good health. Remember, a physical examination, no matter how complete, is only a snapshot in time. Tomorrow things can change, perhaps slowly, perhaps not so slowly. So if there are any changes in the way you feel, be sure to alert your doctor, even if it has only been one week since your physical.

Frequency of Physical Examinations

Many patients are confused about how often they need to have periodic physicals and screening tests when they are healthy and "asymptomatic" (a doctor word for feeling well). Luckily, there are guidelines published by The American Cancer Society and The American Heart Association which give general rules of thumb as to how to manage a good preventive health care plan.

Hint: *These are guidelines only* and are not set in concrete. You and your doctor should decide between you what level of frequency is right for you based upon your family and personal health history, and any risk factors, such as smoking, which may apply to you.

History: Should be taken every five years for ages twenty to sixty, every two-and-a-half years for ages sixty-one to seventy-five, and every year thereafter.

Physical exams vary according to what is being looked for: The newest American Heart Association guidelines have moved away from the annual physical and now call for physicals which thoroughly check out the heart and blood systems every five years until sixty, every two-and-a-half years thereafter until age seventy-five and annually thereafter.

The American Cancer Society recommends an examination for cancers of the thyroid, testicles, prostate, ovaries, lymph nodes and skin every three years until age forty, and then every year thereafter. It also recommends a digital rectal examination for everyone once a year past the age of forty. Women should have their doctors examine their breasts once every three years between the ages of twenty and forty and every year thereafter.

Hint: I repeat, these are only *guidelines.* Your personal physician may wish to see you more often. Also, this *does not apply to children,* who should see their doctors far more frequently. Ask your pediatrician or family care specialist for the "Recommendations for Preventive Health Care of Children and Youth," published by The American Academy of Pediatrics, and discuss with your physician how these guidelines apply to your child, individually.

Pelvic examinations, according to The American Cancer Society, should be taken by all healthy women every three years from the ages of twenty to forty, and once every year thereafter. If you have an abnormal Pap test, you will need to be examined more often.

Blood pressure readings should be obtained by a *healthy* person who shows *no symptoms* of high blood pressure or heart disease, every two-and-a-half to five years until age sixty-one, and then every two-and-a-half years. After age seventy-five, the test should be given annually.

Sigmoidscopies, according to The American Cancer Society, should be administered to both men and women once every three years *after* two normal exams have been given one year apart. This routine should begin at age fifty.

Stool tests should be taken once a year after age fifty.

Mammograms are recommended once between the ages of thirty-five to forty to obtain a baseline and then every one to two years, until age fifty. Thereafter, a woman should receive an annual test.

Blood tests for cholesterol should be taken every five years until age sixty and every two-and-a-half years thereafter, if good baselines have been documented.

Urinalysis should be given every two years or so until the age of forty and approximately every year thereafter.

Chest x-rays are not recommended by The American Cancer Society as a lung cancer screening tool for healthy individuals. The American Heart Association recommends that a baseline x-ray be taken at about the age of forty.

EKGs should be taken for baseline purposes at ages twenty, forty and sixty.

Remember, these are only *general guidelines* and do not constitute the entire range of examinations or screening procedures that are available. Also remember, if you smoke, have abnormal test results, or a health history which indicates that you should receive more frequent exams, these guidelines may not apply in your case. So be sure to *ask your doctor what specific program of preventive care should be established individually for you.*

When Something May Be Wrong

There comes into each of our lives a time when our bodies tell us that there may be a "glitch" in the system that needs to be checked out. Doctors call these glitches "symptoms"; you and I refer to them as "not feeling right."

If a symptom introduces itself to you, what should you do? Obviously, you should call your doctor and discuss it (which is a reason again to have a primary care physician). If you don't have a doctor, stop by an urgent care clinic and meet with one of their doctors, or make an appointment with a primary care physician.

The following is a brief list of symptoms that should cause you to seek immediate medical assistance:

The Seven Warning Signals Of Cancer

- Change in bowel or bladder habits
- A sore that does not heal
- Unusual bleeding or discharge
- Thickening or lump in breast or elsewhere
- Indigestion or difficulty in swallowing
- Obvious change in wart or mole
- Nagging cough or hoarseness

(Reprinted with the permission of The American Cancer Society.)

Remember, the sooner cancer is diagnosed, the better your chances of surviving. So don't refrain from seeing a doctor because you are afraid of what the results will be. Chances are your problem will not be cancer, but if it *is,* it sure won't go away by pretending it's not there.

Symptoms of Heart and Vascular Disease

There are many physical symptoms that might indicate that you have developed heart disease. These include the obvious, like chest pains, to the less expected, such as shortness of breath, sudden shortness of breath at night, palpitations, edema (accumulation of fluid in body cavities or connective tissue), unexplained limping (claudication) and fatigue. Ask your doctor or your local branch of The American Heart Association for further details.

Miscellaneous Maladies

Of course, this book cannot list every physical symptom that should cause you to be concerned enough to contact a doctor. But here are some of the more important ones that should not be ignored:

- Out-of-the-ordinary headaches
- High fever (of 103 degrees or more), or fever that persists more than a few days
- Sudden change in vision
- Seizure or sudden weakness in any arm or leg
- Coughs lasting more than a few days, or coughs associated with shortness of breath, sweating or dizziness

- Chest pain on exertion, or that which is associated with sweating, dizziness or shortness of breath
- Abdominal pain along with a fever or vomiting, or a rapid swelling of the abdomen
- Vomiting blood, or blood in the stool (which may look like tar)
- Swelling in legs or feet
- Anything else that *common sense* tells you is not right

If you experience any of the above, *call your doctor immediately!* It may be nothing, but why take a chance? If your doctor believes your problems need to be looked into, he or she will recommend that you come in to be examined. Or, you may be directed to go to an emergency room or to call the paramedics. You may also be tested, by the tests mentioned above or by even more sophisticated diagnostic tools, such a CT Scan.

If your doctor recommends testing, ask the following questions to make sure the tests are reasonable and worth the time, effort and expense.

Why is this particular test required? Sometimes more than one test can be utilized to obtain similar results. In such cases you may want to see if there is a less expensive or more comfortable alternative.

What are you looking for? Part of giving informed consent is knowing the purpose for a test being given. Also, you should be told what the doctor suspects so that you can obtain information about the suspected condition(s) yourself.

How is it done? Testing is a tough enough process to go through without having to be surprised. Thus, if you are going to be stuck with needles, you have the right to know. If chemicals are going to be introduced into your system, you have the right to know. And, needless to say, if the test requires a trip to the hospital, you should know.

What will I feel during and after the test? Sometimes, like during an x-ray, you will feel nothing. At other times, you may feel some pain or require some form of anesthesia. Whatever the case will be, you have the right to know, including any potential side effects or "after effects" such as exhaustion.

What are the risks? Some tests are virtually risk-free, others are not. You have the right to know if there is any danger involved, and if so, to what degree so that you can make an intelligent decision about whether to proceed.

How much will the procedure cost? When it comes to matters of health, money should not have top priority in our decision-making process. However, you certainly have the right to know what the price will be so that you can make a cost vs. hoped-for benefit analysis about whether to "go for broke" or "fall back ten and punt."

Will my health insurance pay for any of the costs? Pray that the answer to that one is "yes!"

What are the consequences of not doing the test? Part of your basic dignity as a human being is your control over what happens or doesn't happen to your body. This means you have the right to refuse a recommended test if you so desire. (Of course, refusing a doctor's recommendation may be foolhardy, but it certainly is your right.) Just make sure you fully understand the consequences before you say "*Nyet*."

Hint: A major issue in medicine today concerns the issue of diagnostic tests and cost control. Are three tests too many? Is one test enough? What's a patient to do?

Follow the money. If the *profit* to your doctor or medical facility *will come by doing more tests,* your self-protection radar should probably be aimed at making sure you are only given those procedures you absolutely need to effect an accurate diagnosis.

If, on the other hand, *the profit comes from not performing diagnostic tests,* such as with an HMO, don't hesitate to be the squeaky wheel that gets the grease (tests) by insisting that your doctor order the tests which are necessary to come up with an accurate diagnosis. If you don't know what tests there are—*ask!*

NOTES TO THE CHART

When it comes to our own health, doctors are like any other patient. We don't like to take tests, be stuck with needles or undergo physical exams any more than any other patient does. But when the results come back normal—what a happy and wonderful feeling!

Preventive care is a vital part of protecting your own health and vitality. The most important element in this program is a close relationship with your doctor, accompanied by routine physical examinations. Also, if you don't feel well, don't hesitate to call your doctor. That's what he or she is there for.

If your doctor recommends further testing after the routine set, he or she should explain why the test is necessary and what is being looked for. Never be afraid to ask questions. Questions will not only get you the information you are looking for, but will tell the physician whether the information he or she is trying to impart is getting through. One more thing: don't accept vague non-answers when working with a physician. *You have the right to know what is going on.*

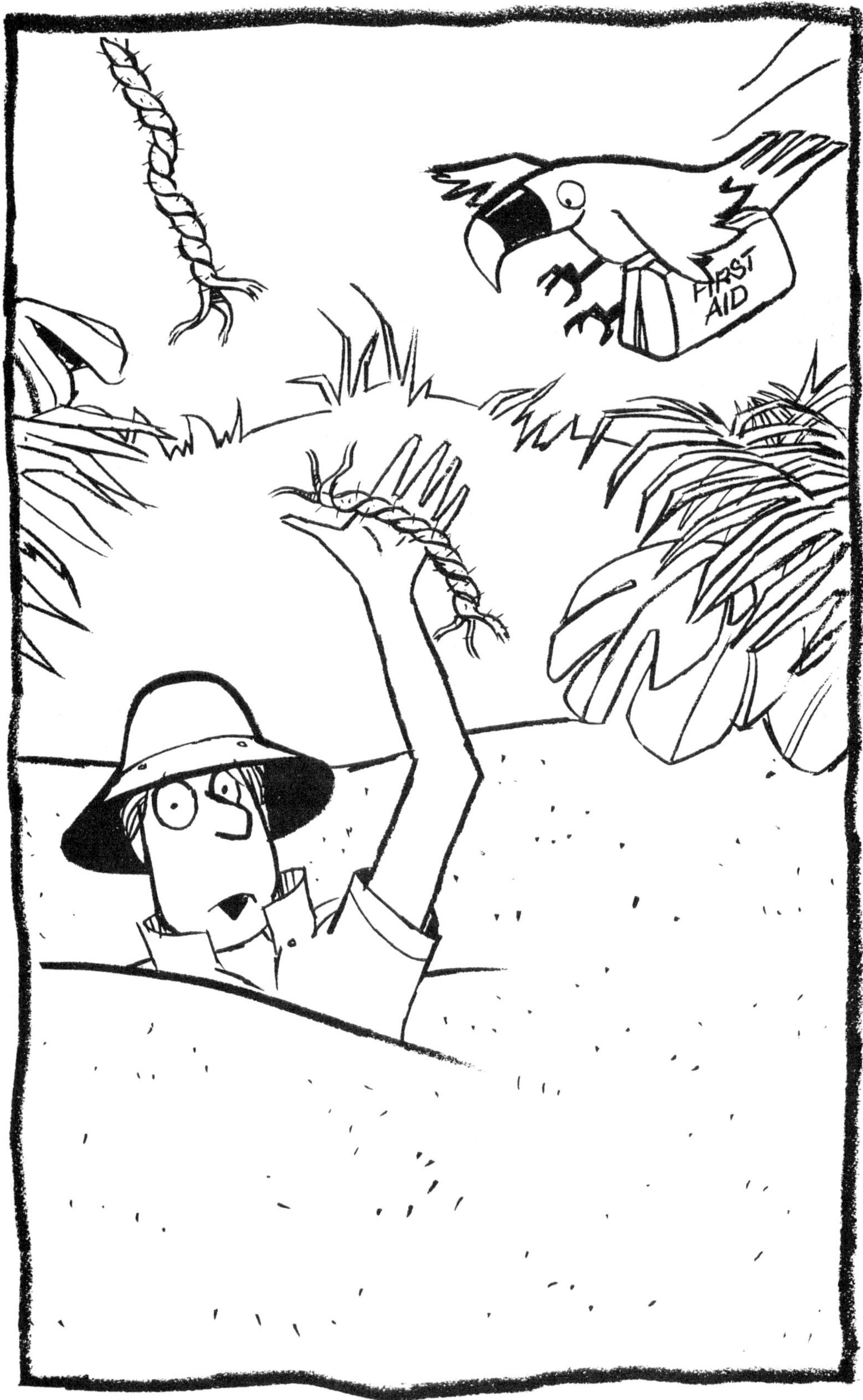
FIRST
AID

·7·

CHAPTER

Help, I Need Somebody

Seeking Emergency Treatment

FADE IN: Hospital Emergency Room, Night: *The camera follows Peter Pillpusher, M.D., the newly appointed chief resident of the graveyard shift, as he enters the E.R. of Soapsud Hospital. As Peter enters, the eyes of every nurse and patient are riveted on the young, handsome doctor with the piercing stare and lantern jaw, especially those of buxom Nurse Bonnie Luscious. Their eyes meet and flash in remembrance of that special night they recently shared when accidentally locked in the hospital pathology lab.*

Peter: *(with suppressed passion)* Nurse, status report, please.

Bonnie tries to maintain a professional demeanor, but her voice cracks as she speaks.

Bonnie: Two accident victims, both stabilized. One heart attack on his way to I.C.U. . . Oh, Peter, why didn't you tell me you were married before . . .

A single tear runs down Bonnie's left cheek. Peter takes her hands in his.

Peter: Do you think I would have allowed you to give me your heart if I had known my wife had survived that avalanche in the Himalayas? What kind of man do you think I am?

Bonnie: If I only knew, Peter. If I only knew.

Suddenly the sound of sirens is heard. An orderly runs up to Peter.

Orderly: Dr. Pillpusher! There's been a shooting! It's Mayor Legree!

Cue the organ music—close up on Peter. He grabs the orderly's shoulders.

Peter: Simon's been shot? Are you sure?

Bonnie reaches out for the distraught Peter.

Peter: Bonnie, what I am going to do? Simon was my best friend until he framed me for the murder of my first wife, Sarah. And now he's been shot and I have to try to save his life. I don't think I can do it. . .

Like this scene, emergency rooms have often provided the perfect setting for movies, books and television programs. After all, the key ingredient of any vehicle of popular entertainment is conflict, and where better to find conflict than in a place where matters of life and death are all part of a day's routine?

But you and I live in the real world where conflict is usually the *last* thing we want to experience. This is especially true in an emergency situation, where quick, competent and effective medical service is the order of the day, not conflict. The best way to avoid conflict in an emergency setting is to understand how the system operates and what you can do as an intelligent health care consumer to make it work efficiently and effectively for you.

• Be Prepared •

The Boy Scout motto "Be prepared" is especially good advice when it comes to handling medical emergencies. After all, if you have made plans in advance as to how you are going to cope with the unexpected, your chances of getting through a crisis unscathed will be greatly enhanced. Here are some common sense points to include in your health emergency preparation agenda.

Locate the best emergency rooms in the areas where you live, work and frequently play. Nearly everyone knows that most hospitals have emergency rooms where medical assistance is available in the event of urgent need. However, many of us do not know that all hospitals do not have emergency rooms staffed around the clock. In fact, some hospitals have no emergency service at all. Thus, the first task of smart health care consumers is to decide in advance where they or their families will go in the event of an emergency. In that way, should the need ever arise, you won't have to stop at a corner gas station to ask for directions to the nearest hospital. (And with all of the self-serve "service" stations around these days, you might have difficulty receiving even *that.*)

Hint: Today, most hospital emergency rooms are staffed by physicians who are board-certified or board-qualified in the specialty of Emergency Medicine. And so, when determining which hospital you will want to take your emergency medical business to, call each hospital under consideration and ask if their E.R. physicians are emergency specialists or whether they are "moonlighting" doctors who mainly practice in other fields.

Hint: Ask your family doctor for the name and location of the best emergency rooms in your area. After all, he or she has the means to know the good ones from the not-so-good ones.

Keep important medical information about yourself on your person at all times. The basic health information that any doctor needs to have in order to treat you effectively may be even more important for the physician to know in a medical emergency. Thus, it is a very good idea to keep a small note card in your wallet or purse which contains the name and telephone number of your PCP, lists your allergies and any medications (along with dosage) you may be taking, and whether you are pregnant. Also, if you happen to suffer from a medical condition, especially one that can render you unconscious, such as diabetes or epilepsy, make sure the card lists that ailment. In that way, if you are rushed to a hospital unconscious, the E.R. doctor will be immediately alerted to your condition when trying to find the cause of your problem.

Hint: You should also list the name and phone number of whom you want contacted in the event of an emergency. This person should probably be a relative or someone who has a power of attorney to give consent for your medical care in the event you are unable to give it yourself. Also, be sure this person has knowledge of your medications and other necessary information, just in case.

Hint: If you are elderly or have a heart condition, it is a good idea to keep a copy of your baseline EKG in your wallet so that any changes could be noted by E.R. personnel.

A Note About MedicAlert:

If you or a loved one have a serious medical condition such as Alzheimer's disease, diabetes, asthma, epilepsy, hypertension or heart disease, or if you are allergic to substances such as the venom of insect stings or penicillin, or if you must take medication such as beta-blockers or steroids, think very seriously about getting a MedicAlert chain or bracelet. For a twenty dollar membership fee you get:

- *A bracelet or necklace with the MedicAlert logo which tells emergency medical personnel that you have a specific health condition that they need to know about.*

- *The back of the bracelet or necklace will list your medical condition and/or medications you take.*

- *A 24-hour hotline provides other medical information which an emergency medical team might require, such as the name and phone number of your doctor and the name and phone number of who should be contacted in an emergency.*

- *A back-up wallet card is also issued which contains the same information.*

For more information about this tax-exempt, nonprofit foundation, write to MedicAlert Foundation International, Turlock, CA 95381-1009, or call toll-free (800) ID-ALERT.

Have consent forms on file with the local emergency room in advance. This can be very important if you are a parent and you will be out of town or otherwise unreachable should your child have a medical emergency while at school. In such cases, visit the emergency room of the hospital to which your child will be taken in an emergency and fill out a consent form in advance. In this way, the doctors will be able to get right to work and won't have to deal with the red tape of obtaining a social worker or court approval prior to rendering medical assistance.

Know the health symptoms that indicate a medical emergency exists. One of the more common reactions to unexpected severe medical difficulties is denial. After all, serious illness reminds us that we are mortal, and who wants to deal with that? Besides, we tell ourselves we will *certainly* have enough advanced notice to allow us to prepare for our final curtain. Wrong. And our refusal to admit this can be the reason we are taken "before our time."

Therefore, it is a good idea to know the symptoms of sudden killers like strokes and heart attacks. In that way, should we ever experience these symptoms, or observe someone else doing so, we will be less likely to deny the potential seriousness of what is going on.

Heart Attack: According to The American Heart Association, the following are symptoms of a heart attack which you ignore literally at the risk of your own life:

• Pressure or pain or a feeling of fullness or squeezing in the center of the chest that lasts two minutes or longer

• Pain spreading to the shoulders, neck or arms. The pain can also originate in any one of these parts.

• Dizziness, a feeling of faintness, sweating, nausea or shortness of breath

Stroke: A stroke is the common name for a physiological event when, because of internal bleeding or clotting, the supply of oxygen and nutrients to the brain is impeded. Here are the symptoms The American Heart Association lists as warning signals of this deadly and debilitating affliction:

• Sudden, temporary weakness or numbness of the face, arm and leg on one side of the body

• Temporary loss of speech, or trouble understanding speech. (A friend of mine had a mild stroke. His symptom was the temporary loss of the ability to read.)

• Temporary dimmed vision or loss of vision, particularly in one eye

• Unexplained dizziness, unsteadiness or falls

Major strokes are often preceded by "little strokes" known as TIAs (transient ischemic attacks) which have similar *short-lived* symptoms. If you suffer from what may be a TIA, go to an E.R. or call your doctor *immediately!* TIAs are warning signs that a full-fledged stroke may be on the way.

If you suffer any of these symptoms, don't wait to see if they will go away, call the paramedics or have someone drive you immediately to the nearest emergency room with a cardiac care unit and let them figure out what's going on.

There are, of course, other situations when you must go to an emergency room. These include:

- Unconsciousness
- Serious injury

- Severe bleeding
- Unexplained drowsiness
- Unexplained seizures
- Severe pain and/or cramping
- Cold sweats or hyperventilation
- Any feeling, no matter how vague or imprecise, that leads you to believe you are experiencing or are about to experience a medical emergency

Regardless of the symptom, if you have a medical problem which you believe requires the assistance of a doctor, your local emergency room is there to help you. And when in doubt, play it safe, or at the very least, give your local E.R. or your doctor a call. Playing it safe is always better than being sorry.

Hint: If you need to see a doctor but feel you are not in a life-threatening situation (such as having a bad cut on the hand), call your own doctor to see if you can be squeezed in. If you can't be seen, you will at least receive useful guidance on the steps to take to solve your medical problem.

Hint: For those in less serious distress, a viable alternative to the local E.R. (which usually requires a lot of waiting) is the "urgent care clinic," which specifically caters to illnesses and injuries which are non-life-threatening, but which nevertheless require immediate medical attention.

The E.R. Experience

I think it is safe to say that emergency rooms are *not* fun places to be in. Patients can be seen everywhere writhing in agony and begging for relief, and that's just over the registration procedures. Or, to misquote Churchill, where else will you find so many being waited on by so few? (Except perhaps at your local Department of Motor Vehicles office.)

Yet, despite their reputations, a well-run emergency room can be an oasis of healing in a desert of medical despair, whose many inconveniences are more than outweighed by the medical relief to be found there. And once explained, even the inconveniences and delays can be seen to have a productive, if irritating, purpose.

JACK AND JILL II: IN THE EMERGENCY ROOM

Most everyone grew up hearing the story of Jack and Jill "going up a hill to fetch a pail of water." But no one knows what happened to them *after* "Jack fell down and broke his crown and Jill came tumbling after." Let's pick up where the story left off, following the pair as they get treatment for their injuries.

Jill: After my tumble I felt a ripping in my left ankle. When I looked over at Jack, he was holding his bleeding head. I limped over to him and he said he felt sick to his stomach and that his back hurt. Luckily, we had our cellular phone in the BMW, so I called the nearby emergency room to let them know we were coming in. The nurse who answered the phone suggested that I call the paramedics because she was worried about Jack's condition.

Except in obviously life-threatening situations such as a shooting or a heart attack (where you should dial 911 or another emergency number), it's usually a good idea to call the emergency room ahead of time to tell them you want to come in. You will probably talk with a "triage nurse" who will ask you about the injured or ill person's symptoms and who will tell you:

• Whether you need to come in (the benefit of any doubts being in favor of coming in, or at the very least, calling your own doctor)

• Whether you can come in as a "walk in" or whether you should call the paramedics

• What to do for the person in need of assistance before you arrive

• What information you need to bring with you to the hospital

• Whether you will be better off (in a minor injury situation) going to a different E.R. or urgent care clinic because they are already "full," thus saving you a potential multi-hour delay in receiving treatment

A call placed before leaving for the hospital also allows the E.R. staff to prepare for your arrival, which can help them serve you more efficiently.

Jack: The first thing I remember after my fall was Jill holding me in her arms and the sound of sirens as the paramedics arrived. Before they took me away, they called the hospital on the radio and told them what was going on. The paramedics were instructed to take special precautions regarding my back. It seemed like forever, but within thirty minutes of my fall, I was on my way to the hospital.

Jill: I felt able to drive, so I followed the ambulance to the hospital. I was told that the hospital Jack was being taken to was a "trauma center."

Paramedics are more than ambulance drivers, they are specially trained medical technicians who work with personnel of the emergency room to begin treatment while you are on the way to the hospital. This includes more than applying first aid—it can involve the delivery of sophisticated medical procedures administered under the radio supervision of a doctor or mobile intensive care nurse located at a hospital "base station," such as starting IVs (intravenous delivery of medication or fluids) or giving injections.

Hint: Some areas do not provide emergency paramedic service, but rather, merely have EMTs—emergency medical technicians. More than just a title separates the two, for EMTs cannot administer medications, cannot start IVs and do not render much more than first aid to their patients. Thus, the difference between being treated by a paramedic and an EMT *could* be the difference between enjoying a full recovery and attending a funeral—your own.

Trauma centers are far more than fancy emergency rooms. They represent an entire emergency network consisting of paramedics, emergency rooms and specially designated hospitals that are dedicated to bringing specialized emergency care to trauma victims within a sixty-minute time period called "the golden hour." Generally, here's how a trauma network operates:

1. A person in need of trauma care is identified. Cases such as falls from a height of fifteen feet or more, gunshot wounds to the trunk of the body, a penetrating head or neck injury and injuries which destabilize the chest wall are typical of those injuries deemed appropriate for trauma care.

2. The paramedics will not bring a trauma victim to the nearest E.R. as they would normally do, but to the nearest trauma care facility (trauma center), so long as that facility is relatively near (usually no longer than twenty minutes away).

3. At the trauma center, the E.R. personnel will test and stabilize the patient, as usually happens in any emergency room. But then something different happens . . .

4. The trauma victim is admitted to the hospital and surgery is immediately performed as needed, so that the corrective treatment occurs within the golden hour.

Designated trauma centers can spring into action this quickly because they have surgeons either in-house or on call within twenty minutes from the hospital, as opposed to a regular hospital which might not have the appropriate surgeon available on such short notice.

Hint: The time saved *does* save lives, but at an expense. The hospitals have to pay the surgeons to be immediately available and thus usually rely on public funding to support their trauma efforts. In many parts of the country, trauma centers are closing down because of inefficient management or insufficient financing (depending, as is usually the case in such controversies, upon whom you are talking to).

Jill: When we arrived at the hospital, Jack was brought through the ambulance entrance to the emergency room, and I was asked to hobble through the ambulatory care entrance. They went right to work on Jack, and asked me about his medical history. There were so many questions. "When was his last tetanus shot? Is he taking medications? What is he allergic to? Who is his doctor? Does he have health insurance?" I will say though, that they went right to work on Jack, and before too long he was out of the emergency room and into surgery, since the x-rays showed that he had a fractured skull.

In potentially life-threatening situations the emergency room medical staff should treat first and ask questions about payment later. (In fact, in many states that is the law.) Also note the breadth of information about a patient that is needed in emergency situations. After all, the patient is a stranger to the emergency room doctor, and the wrong move with the wrong medication could prove disastrous.

Jill: As soon as I knew Jack was in good hands, I remembered how much my ankle hurt. I noticed that it was badly swollen and I asked for treatment. I was interviewed by a nurse and told that I would probably have to wait "a few minutes" before the doctor could see me. I was asked to register, a process which took about fifteen minutes. After thirty minutes I asked when I would be seen. I was told that another ambulance had come in with a heart attack victim and that all of the other beds were taken. Then a woman came in with a little girl who had a very high fever. She was seen immediately, while I ended up waiting over an hour before I was seen by a doctor. Boy, was I ever mad.

Patients who seek assistance at an emergency room are not seen "first come, first serve." They don't take numbers like in an ice cream shop. Rather, E.R.s operate on a *"most in need,* first serve" basis. Jill had to wait because her condition was less serious than that of others who were seeking assistance at the same emergency room at the same time.

When a patient comes to an emergency room, he or she will be interviewed by a nurse to determine the extent of his or her medical need. Those in the greatest distress are seen first, while those with more minor complaints are seen later. This process of selecting and giving priority care to those patients in greatest need of assistance is called the "triage" process, which literally means "to sort."

Hint: The questions you will be asked in the triage process will include queries regarding your health history as well as your immediate symptoms. All of the information that is taken down is put on your chart and used later by the doctor when seeking to treat or diagnose your problem. So, you see, the time is *not* wasted. In fact, the triage system allows the emergency room to run at maximum efficiency.

The hospital staff did make a mistake by being vague when Jill asked how long she would have to wait for treatment (not an unreasonable request). As one doctor put it, the "art" of running an emergency room is in "managing the wait." This means that you have the right to be told a best estimate of the length of time you will have to wait before you can be seen by medical personnel. And if it looks like the wait will exceed the estimate, you have the right to be told that too, as well as the reason for the added delay (such as, "A heart attack patient just arrived").

Hint: If you have been asked to wait and your distress becomes more acute (that's Doctorese for "you feel sicker"), definitely *speak up.* Your spot on the triage list may need to be reconsidered.

You should also try to be understanding if someone with a different problem of the same severity is seen before you. After all, an emergency room must be prepared for all comers, and so may have limited facilities for each specific problem. (For example, there may be only one area equipped to handle ear, nose and throat problems.) In Jill's case, a sick child was seen before she was because that child needed an ice bath and the space designated for that treatment was immediately available, while the bed Jill would later use while her ankle was being examined was occupied by someone with a more serious injury than hers.

Jill: When I was taken back into the treatment room, a nurse took my temperature, blood pressure and pulse. I was left alone for about ten minutes and then a doctor came in and looked at my ankle. He said it didn't look broken but decided I should have an x-ray. I figured that while I had the doctor there, I'd ask him to check my tonsils, since I had a sore throat for two days. That quack said I should call my own doctor about tonsils because he was "too busy to deal with that now!" Can you believe it?

Many people make the mistake of using emergency room doctors as their primary care physicians. This is a bad idea for several reasons:

Training: As discussed above, emergency room physicians are specialists who are trained in emergency medicine. They are *not* primary care physicians and don't pretend to be.

Purpose: The emergency room is not designed to provide long-term treatment, but is designed primarily to provide preliminary care in order to stabilize the patient so that appropriate medical treatment can be obtained elsewhere. (Of course, there are times when the treatment received in an emergency room is the only medical care required.) A patient who is seen in an emergency room will thereafter either be released, admitted to the hospital for further treatment, transferred to another hospital for even further treatment or be released and possibly advised to get further treatment. (Although there may be some follow-up care given under limited circumstances.)

Scope: When you are being evaluated at an E.R., only those medical matters which are urgent will be dealt with. Thus, the emergency room doctor who cares very much about your chest pains will probably give short shrift to your questions about the arthritis in your elbow.

Tests: A patient who is treated in an emergency situation may undergo either more or less diagnostic testing than would be received from their primary care physicians. More, in the sense that an E.R. doctor who does not know a patient's history may order tests that would be seen as unnecessary if the doctor had known the patient, and less since secondary problems might not be dealt with at all.

Cost: Treatment at an emergency room is more expensive than treatment from a primary care physician—sometimes more than twice as expensive.

Hint: Try to limit your use of hospital emergency rooms to truly serious injuries or illnesses. Your own doctor should be able to treat you for the less serious matters, or at the very least, refer you to another physician for immediate treatment. And, of course, matters that require long-term care are inappropriate for the emergency room unless a major crisis flares up requiring immediate attention.

Jill: After I had my x-rays, I was told that my ankle *was* broken. A cast was put on and I was told I should consult with an orthopedist. I told them I needed the name of one and I was given the name of someone to call and told to see the doctor within two days. They also told me the orthopedist would receive copies of my records. I was given "crutch training," some paperwork, a prescription for pain pills, and I was released. The entire process took about two hours.

When you leave the emergency room, you should be told what your diagnosis was, or in some cases, what it wasn't, and you should receive specific instructions, preferably in writing, about what to look for by way of complications, how to handle yourself and what you should do in terms of follow-up care.

Two months later Jack and Jill were both almost completely recovered. The speed with which Jack was treated was credited with saving his life. Jill didn't like the doctor the emergency room had referred her to, so she had her PCP help her find one that suited her better. Jack did have something of a fuss with his HMO insurance plan over the timing of his transfer to their hospital facility. But that's another story. . .

Potpourri: More To Know About The E.R.

Here are some final notes about emergency rooms and the process of emergency care.

When possible have a friend or loved one come with you to the emergency room. After all, you may be in too much misery to comprehend fully everything that is happening, and you will need someone who can help you put the pieces together later on. Besides, it never hurts to have someone you trust monitoring your care to make sure all is done correctly.

Make sure you or your "monitor" understand and approve of all diagnostic testing and treatment. Overtesting does occur in an emergency room context, since the E.R. doctor knows that there may be a malpractice lawyer looking over his or her shoulder. If you feel this is a problem, tell the doctor to confer with your PCP to see if the tests can be delayed until your own doctor can do them. Also remember that your right to give informed consent still applies except under the most critical circumstances.

If you have further medical difficulty after receiving treatment, call the emergency room to discuss it. Sometimes patients have continuing difficulty after being treated at an E.R., but don't call to discuss it. Anytime a problem has arisen with the illness or injury after emergency care, call the emergency room or your own doctor! After all, when it comes to your health, silence is *not* golden.

Always get your primary care physician involved. Be sure to have the emergency room call your doctor to see if he or she wants to be in charge of your care and to coordinate your treatment. Also, make sure your own doctor receives copies of all of your emergency room medical records.

If you are a member of an HMO, tell the emergency room personnel. As we discussed earlier, when you join an HMO, you agree to use their facilities and doctors exclusively except in an emergency. If you seek medical care at a non-HMO emergency room, and don't obtain prior approval from your plan, the emergency or urgent care you receive may well be on you.

Let the E.R. know how you feel about the care you received. The only way that a hospital really knows if the services they provide are adequate is if they hear from their patients. So, if you were happy with your care, let them know. If not, complain in writing, listing the specific problems you had with the facility. Send your letter to the medical director of the emergency room with a copy to the hospital administrator.

Notes To The Chart

Things have changed since I moonlighted in an emergency room during my internal medicine residency. At that time I remember losing some of the little sleep I did get worrying over running into an emergency that was beyond my ability to handle.

Fortunately, life in the emergency room has changed. Today, specialists in emergency medicine staff most of the country's emergency rooms, which has raised the level of care that these important service facilities can offer. In my capacity as a primary care physician and as a sub-specialist in infectious disease, I have had an opportunity to watch these fine physicians in action. To say the least, I have been very, very impressed.

This chapter has accurately described what you can expect to encounter should you have to visit an emergency room. Remember, an E.R. is designed to handle emergencies, and so the overhead costs to the hospital are higher, which are in turn reflected in your bill. Thus, if your medical problem is not an emergency, call your own doctor before you go to the hospital E.R. He or she will probably be able to squeeze you in, which will allow you to receive more personalized care at less cost.

One last piece of advice: if you are ill during the week, contact your own doctor. Otherwise, if you wait until the weekend to seek help, the E.R. may be your only source of immediate medical care.

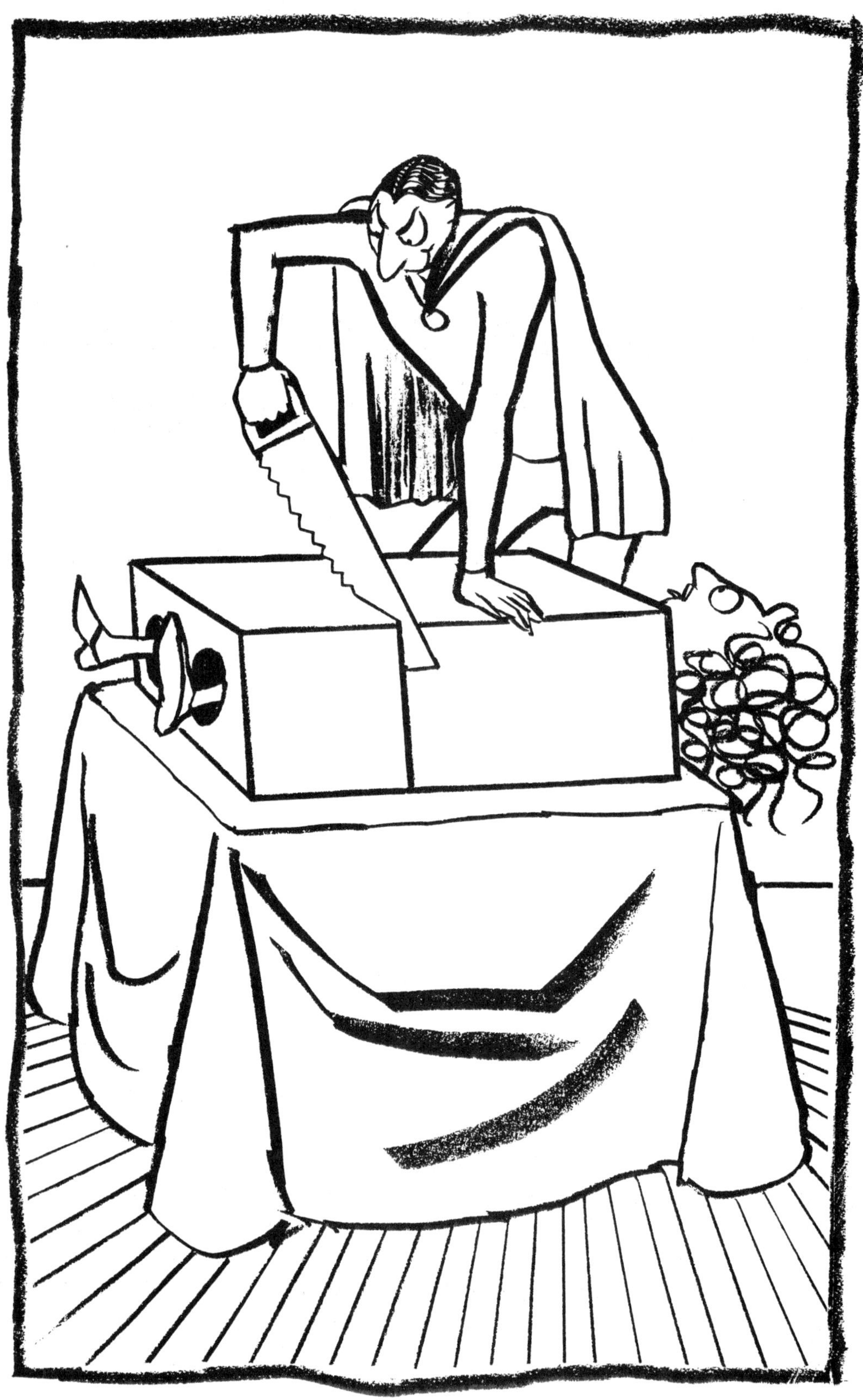

·8·

CHAPTER

To Cut Or Not To Cut, That Is The Question

· The World Of Surgery ·

"Scalpel."
"Scalpel, Doctor."
"Sponge."
"Sponge, Doctor."
"Forceps . . . Forceps . . . I said forceps, Nurse!"
"Forceps."
"Carefully, carefully . . . Got it!"
"Doctor, you're a genius!"
"I know."

Unfortunately, this over-dramatized scene, obviously depicting a surgery, contains about as much information as most of us know about this "glamour" field of the medical arts. In other words, next to nothing.

Surgery is a simple word, really, but one that fills most of us with a sense of dread—especially if we hear the word preceded by the phrase, "I'm sorry, but I'm afraid you are going to have to have . . ." Yet, despite its real and imagined dangers, modern surgery is a major medical lifesaver that can often be the difference between a life of quality or a life of illness, or even any life at all. And since into every life "a little surgery must fall" (either personally or to a loved one or friend), the more that is known about the process, the less likely the chance that mistakes will be made.

Deciding to have surgery is not like deciding that the time has come to buy a new stereo. I mean, no one wakes up and says, "Gee, I think I'll go and have some surgery today!" Yet, some patients handle this important life decision almost that casually, as if the only say they have in the matter is over which robe they should bring with them to the hospital.

When it comes to surgery, patients have as much right to be at the cause of their treatment, and have as many decisions to make regarding it, as they do in every other area of medical care. And since any surgery carries with it the potential for serious and even devastating consequences, patient power is never more important than here.

Choosing A Surgeon

Surgeries generally fall into broad categories, emergency and elective. Emergency surgeries are those procedures which must be done *right now* to save life or limb, no "ifs, ands or buts" about it. In such emergencies, you may have no say at all over who performs your operation (unless you were already planning surgery and the emergency arose before you could get to it). I mean, if you've been brought to a hospital with collapsed lungs from an automobile accident, no one is going to take the time to ask the surgeon on call whether or not he or she is board-certified.

Luckily, most operations are elective, giving you a much broader opportunity to make choices as to the selection of the surgeon and even the procedure itself. For our purposes, an elective surgery is one that can range from not medically necessary, such as cosmetic surgery, to surgery that *must* be done, just not this very second. As a result of this "luxury of time" (which can be short or long, depending on the individual circumstances), the patient usually does have the opportunity to exercise some control over his or her own destiny.

Check Out The Surgeon's Skills

Most patients see a surgeon because their primary care physician has told them that surgery is a step that must be taken. Thus, most patients are not "walk-ins," but have been specifically referred by another doctor.

That does not mean that you must select the surgeon your doctor recommends. After all, some physicians refer on the basis of who they play tennis with (and, I suppose, on who won the match). Thus, while you should place great weight on your doctor's recommendation, you should also be very careful in your selection process. After all, you want to *get the best.* That process starts with a check of the surgeon's medical credentials and experience.

Is the surgeon board certified? As discussed earlier, board certification tells you that the surgeon has passed his or her residency and passed tests designed to measure clinical and medical knowledge. A general surgeon's residency lasts for five years, so you can see that by the time surgeons become board-qualified, they will have spent a large chunk of time in operating rooms; this is especially true if they are board certified.

What area is the board certification or qualification in? A surgeon who took his or her residency in vascular surgery and not general surgery may not have the skills to operate adequately on a kidney, just as a surgeon who is board-certified in general surgery should probably decline to perform delicate surgery on the aorta (one of the major arteries leading from the heart). So make sure that the residency and board certification is relevant to your medical problem.

How many surgeries such as the one you may need has the surgeon performed? You know what they say, "Practice makes perfect." That sage advice is particularly appropriate when it comes to surgery, since most operations are delicate and intricate procedures requiring an artisan's skills—skills that grow with experience. Thus, if you are going to allow somebody to operate on you, you definitely want that person to be experienced in the same type of procedure you are going to have. If you ask a prospective surgeon how many surgeries such as yours he or she performs a month and the answer is "three a year," that may not be the surgeon to select unless the operation is a rare one, in which case make sure that surgeon has sufficient experience in the procedure to do the job well.

Is the surgeon a Fellow of the American College of Surgeons (F.A.C.S.)? The American College of Surgeons is a voluntary organization limited to physicians who devote themselves to surgical practice. The college demands certain standards of its members (fellows), which is contained in its pledge of membership. These standards include: a commitment to place the welfare of the patient above all else, a promise to continually seek to increase their education and skills, and a pledge not to engage in fee-splitting. The requirements of membership constitute a screening process which alerts you that a surgeon who is F.A.C.S. has met the following minimum standards:

- Graduation from an approved medical school

• Board certification in a relevant specialty (with certain limited exceptions)

• Five years of uninterrupted surgical practice in *one location,* intended as permanent, *after* completion of formal training. Thus a fellow will have been a surgeon for a minimum of five years after completion of his or her surgical residency.

• A current staff appointment at a surgical hospital related to the applicant's surgical specialty

• Applicants are required to submit a recent twelve-month surgical list which is reviewed by the Credentials Committee. This peer review is an important aspect of the value of the college to medical consumers and covers both medical competence and ethical fitness.

If you select a member of The American College of Surgeons as your surgeon, it does not guarantee that the surgeon is good, but it probably improves the odds. For a list of F.A.C.S. surgeons who practice in your area, write:

The American College of Surgeons
Office of Public Information
55 East Erie St.
Chicago, IL 60611-2797

Is the surgeon a member of any other voluntary medical societies? There are many other medical associations in the United States that support physicians in their profession by way of continuing education, peer review and recognition of merit. Many of these professional groups also provide educational materials for consumers and strive to maintain a high level of professional competence and integrity among their members. For example, there is a medical society called The American Academy of Facial Plastic and Reconstructive Surgery, which is the world's largest organization of surgeons who specialize in facial plastic surgery. In order to be a member, a surgeon must:

• Be board-certified in head or neck surgery, ophthalmology, plastic surgery or dermatology

• Have graduated from a residency training program approved by the academy

• Be a member of the American College of Surgeons

• Have proven clinical experience and expertise in facial plastic surgery
In that regard, an applicant must submit thirty-five detailed cases per-

formed in the previous year for peer review.

The Academy even has a toll-free consumer hotline to assist patients with questions about facial plastic surgery (1-800-332-FACE).

Most associations have referral services, require continuing education and provide peer review procedures, which help keep the quality of service high. Ask your doctor if there is a surgical society similar to this academy in the discipline you may have need of, and then contact it for consumer information or for referrals.

Does the surgeon have a position in any hospitals? If a hospital has thought enough of your surgeon's clinical skills to appoint him or her "Chief of Staff" or "Chief of _____ Surgery," it may indicate that the hospital administration and other surgeons have been impressed with his or her skills. Of course, it could also mean nothing more than that the surgeon is a good politician, but if you add board certification to F.A.C.S. along with a staff appointment, well, that surgeon begins to look really solid. (For more details on choosing a doctor, please refer back to Chapter 2.)

Discuss Your Case

Before making the final decision about whether to submit to surgery, you should obviously discuss the matter with the surgeon you decide to consult and with your primary care physician. Here are some of the issues that should be covered:

• **Can surgery be avoided?** Just because your physical condition forces you to consult with a surgeon, that doesn't mean that you will necessarily have to "go under the knife." Part of your surgeon's job is to see whether there are any alternatives to an operation and, if so, work with your PCP or other specialist to pursue them.

> **Hint:** Sometimes the referral to a surgeon is for invasive diagnostic tests rather than "traditional" surgery itself. With regard to these procedures, the same questions should apply.

• **If surgery is indeed recommended, what are the reasons for the recommendation?** The serious step of recommending surgery is not one that is taken lightly by surgeons. Specific indications (objective findings) should be present, which the surgeon and your PCP consider crucial in making the determination that surgery is the way to go. These findings are not state secrets; rather, they should be discussed fully with you in a way that you can understand.

• **What are the expected benefits of the procedure?** Doctors don't just operate on people to see what will happen, they have a specific patient benefit in mind. Be sure you are clear what the specific benefit(s) is in your case before agreeing to proceed. After all, why get a scar for nothing?

• **What will happen if I don't have surgery?** Many elective surgeries seek to repair conditions that cause discomfort but which are not dangerous to life or limb. Others seek to prevent potentially life-threatening situations from developing by "cutting" them off at the pass. (Pardon the pun.) Thus be sure to cover the expected consequences of electing not to proceed before making your decision.

• **What are the risks associated with the surgery?** Every surgery, I repeat, *every surgery* has some element of risk attached to the procedure. It may come from the anesthesia, the threat of aspiration (vomiting and then breathing the material into your lungs, causing a potentially deadly pneumonia), infection or the loss of blood, just to name a few. Your surgeon must, as part of his or her duty to receive your informed consent, tell you about the major risks attendant to the surgery and recovery. (You may not want to hear it, but hear it you must, or the *surgeon* will be hearing from the hospital, hearing from the malpractice insurance company and, if things go wrong, probably hearing from your lawyer.)

Hint: Deciding on surgery is always a balancing test—is the pain, inconvenience and potential danger worth the hoped-for benefits? Thus, if a patient has a disease as deadly as colon cancer, the overall prognosis without surgery, i.e., death, justifies the very major and potentially life-saving surgery of a colostomy. On the other hand, an older person with a weak heart might not want to accept the risks of correcting a limp which is no danger to his or her physical health.

Get A Second Opinion

Second opinions are usually a good idea, especially when it comes to borderline situations or operations such as hysterectomies where studies have shown that some unnecessary operations have been performed. After all, surgery is a very serious business and it always helps to be sure. Besides, as we've already discussed, many insurance companies insist that a second opinion be obtained or they will only pay reduced benefits.

When getting a second opinion, have your previous doctors make all of the tests which have been taken available to the second doctor so that you don't have to undergo the unnecessary time and expense of repeating the test procedures. Also, don't be offended if the second doctor doesn't spend as much time with you as your first one did. His or her job is not to start from scratch but to give you another opinion on the proper course of treatment.

If your PCP, your surgeon and the second-opinion physician all agree that the operation should proceed, it's going to be pretty tough to say no, although that is certainly your right. If they disagree, you may even want a third opinion. But sooner or later you are going to have to decide.

If you say, "It's a go," your job as a patient has only just begun.

• Selecting Your Team •

There's a lot more to undergoing surgery than selecting your surgeon and making a date for the big day. You need to make sure that every member of the medical team who will be responsible for your care is part of the best group of professionals available. After all, even the best pitcher isn't going to win games if the defense can't catch the ball. Likewise, the best surgeon may not do the best job if he or she doesn't have a support team who won't drop the ball.

The Date

The first decision that will have to be made is when the surgery will take place. Some surgeries must be done right away and thus your options may be limited to deciding whether to be operated at 6:00 A.M. or at 8:30 A.M. However, many surgeries are not urgent and you may be given the luxury of planning the procedure around your life. Thus, you may wish to postpone the procedure until you can get off work for some vacation time or until that big project is finished. Whatever the case, discuss your time considerations with your surgeon and PCP so that they can be balanced against your health needs, and an appropriate date can be selected.

Hint: If you are likely to have to receive transfusions of blood, ask your surgeon if you can safely postpone the surgery until such time as you have been able to store your own blood to be given back to you during the procedure. In this way you can be sure that you won't be given somebody else's medical problem, such as hepatitis or AIDS, during the operation. (Although I feel duty-bound to emphasize that the Red Cross blood supply is almost 100% clean of the AIDS virus.)

The Place

It used to be that nearly all but the most trivial surgical procedures were performed in a hospital. Now, with the insurance companies and Medicare seeking to cut costs whenever and wherever possible, there is a much greater push for outpatient surgery. In other words, many surgeries are now performed on a walk-in—walk-out basis, either in the surgeon's office, an ambulatory surgical center or a hospital.

But how do you know whether you are being sent to the appropriate locale for surgery based on your own health needs? That matter should be discussed thoroughly with both your surgeon and primary care physician. Here are some aspects of the question to look at:

What kind of anesthesia will be required? The more powerful the anesthetic, the more likely you will have to be hospitalized due to the possibility of complications, although that certainly isn't the sole criteria for deciding where to be operated upon.

What is the nature of the procedure? Obviously a triple bypass heart operation will require hospitalization, while the removal of an inflamed ingrown toenail probably will not. But since most procedures fall in between those two extremes, you should make sure that the level of seriousness or difficulty of the procedure is matched by the safety of the location where the operation will be performed.

What is the general state of your health? If you are young and vital and your operation is relatively minor, such as a hernia repair, you can probably safely have your operation at a surgical center or at a hospital on an outpatient basis. However, the same surgery being performed on a seventy-eight-year-old man with a history of diabetes and severe heart problems may require hospitalization, not because of the nature of the surgery itself but because of the greater likelihood of serious complications. The less healthy you are generally, the more a hospitalization may be indicated. Again, discuss these matters with your doctors and be prepared to fight your insurance company, which may try to squeeze you into a health care box into which you do not fit.

Remember, the better the location for the surgery is prepared for complications, both with regard to equipment and personnel, the better your chances of escaping complications unscathed should such difficulties arise. Don't allow non-medical considerations to dictate where your surgery will take place if there is any way to prevent it.

When your surgeon makes a recommendation as to where the surgery will take place, ask him or her, "*Why* that particular facility or hospital?"

One hopes the answer will have to do with the quality of the anesthesiologists, other surgical support personnel and the nature of the facility itself, but regardless of the reason given, always check out the reputation of the place with your PCP and others who may be "in the know" beforehand. Remember, it is *your* body and *your* health that we are talking about.

Hint: Sometimes surgeons and other doctors invest in ambulatory surgical centers. If your surgeon recommends that your surgery be performed in a such a place, ask whether he or she has a financial connection with the facility. A "yes" answer will not disqualify the place, but you do have the right to know. Also, if you believe that a different location than the one recommended by the surgeon is more appropriate for you and the surgeon gets angry or hostile instead of seeking to address your concerns, your self-defense radar system should start ringing bells and sounding sirens.

Hint: Sometimes you will be forced to have your surgery at a certain place regardless of its quality because of contractual commitments between your insurance company and the facility. At such times, if you and your doctor feel strongly that the choice of facilities could adversely affect the outcome, see if you and your doctor can talk your insurance company into bending the rules. Otherwise, you may have to decide between having your medical bills paid for and obtaining the best care possible.

The Anesthetic and the Anesthesiologist

An important member of your surgical team, in many ways as important as the surgeon, is the anesthesiologist. In addition to administering the drugs that kill pain, this highly trained physician is in charge of *keeping you alive and healthy* during surgery.

Despite the importance of the anesthesiologist's function, the choice of which one to use may be out of your hands and even out of the hands of your surgeon, at least when it comes to in-hospital procedures. That's because most anesthesiologists work on a contract basis with hospitals, which make the assignments rather than the surgeon. This means that the quality of doctor you get will be based on the quality of the doctors who work out of your hospital and on "the luck of the draw."

Here are some suggestions to help you maintain some control over your own anesthesia:

Ask your surgeon if there are any anesthesiologists whom he or she believes to be superior in the type of procedure you will undergo. (Don't forget, anesthesiologists often get compartmentalized just like doctors do.) If your surgeon tells you, "Dr. Drugem is the best one I've ever worked with," ask your surgeon to request specifically Dr. Drugem. Some hospital administrators may not like the inconvenience that may cause them, but you're in their hospital not for their convenience but for *your health.*

Speak with the anesthesiologist assigned to you before the surgery and discuss what your anesthetic is going to be. Usually, anesthesia is administered under one of the following broad categories:

• Local Block—A limited area of the body is made numb, such as when a dentist gives you a shot of novocaine to deaden one side of your mouth. There is no direct involvement of the brain in local anesthetics. Local blocks are frequently given without an anesthetist present.

• Regional Block—The anesthesiologist introduces drugs into an entire nerve, thus deadening a whole region of the body. The patient does not lose consciousness and the drugs administered do not directly affect the brain.

• General Anesthesia—The patient is rendered unconscious by drugs which *do* impact upon the brain. Frequently referred to by patients as being "put to sleep," this state of unconsciousness is not the same as sleep because the patient cannot be aroused until an antidote is given or the effect of the drugs wears off.

• General Anesthesia with Intubation—The patient is not only rendered unconscious, but is *paralyzed* with a distant cousin of the famous poison, curare. As a result of the paralysis, an endotracheal tube is placed in the patient's mouth and throat and the patient is put on a respirator so that breathing can be accomplished. This type of anesthesia must be used, for example, with all abdominal surgeries, as the surgeon needs to have the abdominal muscles relaxed if he or she is going to be able to do the job. Thus, a procedure like a "tummy tuck," which may sound simple and easy, requires this very involved type of anesthesia. (An endotracheal tube will also be put in during surgeries in which it is suspected that the patient may have eaten prior to the operation, because it protects against aspiration.) The use of an endotracheal tube can give the patient a sore throat and/or chipped teeth or cut lips. Of course, it can and does save lives.

Generally speaking, the less serious the anesthesia, the safer for the patient. Thus, it is a good idea to get by with as "light a dose" as possible based on your health history, present illness, risk factors and the procedure involved, since the lighter the anesthetic, the less chance of complications. (As with the rest of medicine, the exact course of action you and your doctors decide upon will be a matter of balancing risk versus benefit.) Of course there are surgeries where you have no choice, but all of this should be discussed ahead of time with the anesthesiologist, as should the risks attendant to your anesthesia as part of your right to give your informed consent.

At one time, a patient was admitted to the hospital the day before surgery, when he or she would meet and discuss the anesthesia with the anesthesiologist the night before the surgery. Today, many insurance companies require that admissions be on the same day as surgery. Despite this fact, you should still make an effort to meet the anesthesiologist beforehand so that you can get a feel for the doctor and discuss any concerns you might have. You should also tell the anesthesiologist of any previous health problems and about how your body reacted to previous anesthetics. Thus, if you threw up for two days after a previous surgery, bring that to the attention of the anesthesiologist. If the previous medical team had a hard time reviving you, tell the anesthesiologist. Likewise, if everything worked like clockwork the last time, let the anesthesiologist know. After all, he or she is the doctor responsible for keeping you alive as well as out of pain during the surgery.

Hint: If your surgery is in an outpatient clinic (or if anesthesia has made you vomit before), the biggest danger to you may be aspiration. What many insurance companies or medical facilities may not want you to know is that there are drugs which can be administered which have the effect of emptying the stomach, thereby almost eliminating the chances of aspiration. These drugs are expensive and therefore are not often given routinely, but as we all can agree, your health is more important than a corporation's bottom line. Ask your doctor or anesthesiologist about whether he or she recommends that you receive this medication prior to surgery.

Find out what you can expect to feel when the anesthetic wears off. Part of understanding what is going to happen to your body is knowing how the anesthesia will affect it. General anesthesia, for example, can cause vomiting. If you know that and wake up feeling nauseated, it won't scare you as it might if you did not know that it is a common side effect. You should also ask what to look out for if something is wrong, so that you will know to alert the medical personnel that you might be in trouble.

Ask about the cost. Your anesthesiologist will bill you directly. His or her services *are not included* in the surgeon's or hospital's bills. Anesthesiologists generally bill according to a formula which works like this: The American Society of Anesthesiology assigns each type of procedure a number based on difficulty and risk. The anesthesiologist chooses his or her start-up fee, say fifty dollars. The number assigned to the procedure is multiplied by the fee for a total start-up fee (i.e., 3 × $50 = $150). After that, you are also billed for the time the surgery takes, usually in increments of fifteen minutes. Thus a procedure that's rated a three, which took two hours at a time billing of, let's say, $200 per hour, would cost $550 (i.e., 3 × $50 + 2 × $200 = $550). Your anesthesiologist should be able to give you an estimate of costs, insurance coverage and the balance, if any, that you will owe.

Hint: While anesthesiologists are a specialty unto themselves with their own boards and residency programs, some procedures such as pediatric cases or neurological procedures require extra training. Thus, if your operation is one that is so specialized, do your best to obtain an anesthesiologist who has special training in your area of need.

The Assistant Surgeon

Not too many people think about the assistant surgeon when they need an operation. They should. The assistant surgeon can be a vital piece in the successful operation puzzle, serving as a back-up to the surgeon, as an extra pair of hands and eyes, and perhaps most importantly, as an extra brain in the event quick decisions must be made or difficulties arise. Thus, the assistant surgeon is every bit as important as the co-pilot of a jet liner—you can probably survive without one, unless . . .

The problem is, a lot of doctors are acting as assistant surgeons who do not have the same surgical qualifications as the surgeon. Typically, patients want their primary care physician to assist despite the fact that they may have very limited surgical experience. At such times, instead of having two full heads in the surgical suite, there may only be one-and-one-half heads or even one-and-one-quarter. And even though you know and trust your PCP, you need *expertise* in the surgical arena, not a sympathetic hand to hold. Besides, once you're "under," you probably won't know who's in the room anyway.

Keeping the above in mind, it is in your best interest as a patient to *insist that the assistant surgeon have qualifications equal to that of the surgeon.* It won't cost you one penny more, since the assistant receives a fee based on a fixed percentage of the surgeon's charges, typically twenty to twenty-five percent. Since you can have two board-certified surgeons for the same price as a board-certified surgeon and a primary care physician, why not fly first class? (And here you thought there were no bargains left in medicine.)

Hint: Surgeons sometimes get pressure from referring doctors to allow them to assist. If *you* insist that the assistant surgeon be a board-certified surgeon, you will not only help yourself but you may be taking a lot of pressure off of the surgeon to accept a less qualified doctor in the operating room.

• Full Speed Ahead •

Now that you are ready for the big event, there are just a few more things to clarify before you take a deep breath and tell your surgeon to "go to it."

What is the surgery going to cost? You have the right to know ahead of time approximately what the surgery is going to cost. Your surgeon should be able to tell you his or her fees and the fees that will be owed the assistant surgeon. The anesthesiologist or the surgeon should be able to give you a ballpark figure for those services, leaving only the hospital expenses. Those fees may be less predictable, since hospitals usually charge for everything you use while admitted, except for the toilet paper, and I wouldn't be surprised if some charge for that—probably by the square. (This should not apply in an HMO setting.)

What does the fee I pay the surgeon pay for? When you pay a surgeon to perform surgery, you usually get the preoperative care, the surgery and some follow-up care included in the price. Ask your surgeon exactly how much of each you are entitled to for the price so that you don't receive any unexpected and unpleasant post-surgical financial complications. (This should also not apply in an HMO setting.)

What will be happening step-by-step? Everyone fears surgery. However, the worst fear of all is the fear of the unknown, so ask your surgeon what you can expect to happen every step of the way. The following is a scenario of a typical surgery, from the night before through the post-surgery care. (Your experience may vary.)

• **Preparation:** The night before surgery, you will probably meet your anesthesiologist and get to know him or her as a person and discuss your anesthesia. This is your chance to ask any questions you may have about the anesthesia and the anesthesiologist's job. You should also be sure to tell the anesthesiologist of any health problems you have had or problems with previous anesthesia. Your primary care physician is likely to stop by, and you will probably be given a sleeping pill to allow you to get some sleep.

• **Pre-Surgery:** Bright and early the next morning you will be awakened (and this will be a morning that you wish you could sleep late) and transferred to a gurney for a free ride to the surgical suite (just think of it as a poor man's Disneyland). On the way, you will probably receive a shot that will make you forget your troubles and put a smile on your face. (This is not anesthesia but a sedative to calm you.)

Hint: Try to have your surgery scheduled for first thing in the morning. After all, when you are the first in line there is far less chance of a delay.

First stop will be a holding area where the nurses check and double-check who you are and what specific procedure you are going to receive. If you are in a large hospital you will not be alone. The room may be filled with other patients on gurneys just like you. You may be on hold for about thirty minutes, but the time is well spent since the system acts as a failsafe to make sure that you don't have a kidney removed when you thought you were only going to "lose" a cataract.

Finally, you will be wheeled into the surgical suite and the next thing you know . . .

• **Post-Surgery:** You will be taken to the Recovery Room. Here, specially trained nurses will monitor your vital signs and breathing as you come out from under the anesthesia. After you have cleared that hurdle, you will be brought to your next destination, which may be the ICU (intensive care unit), the intermediate care unit or back to your own room to begin the process of recovery. (The ICU is filled with sophisticated monitoring and life-saving equipment and has a patient-to-nurse ratio of no more than two to one. Intermediate Care, as the name implies, has a higher patient-to-nurse ratio and costs about $300 less per day on average.)

Hint: If your surgery is serious, do your best to have it performed at a hospital known for doing major procedures since its ICU will more than likely be staffed by better trained personnel who are more familiar with the problems that can arise after a major surgery.

What can I expect to feel during the recovery period? Every recovery takes time, sometimes more and sometimes less. Every recovery has its ups and downs as well, and you have the right to know what to expect specifically regarding yours. Will you be in pain and, if so, for how long? Must you stay in bed or should you try to become active as soon as possible? Will you need pain pills? What are the warning signs that all is not going according to plan? When can you resume normal activities? The answers to these and other questions will keep you at the "cause" of your own life and make the sometimes frustrating road back to health a little easier to travel.

How will my hospital care be handled? You should be seen and your recovery should be monitored on a daily basis by either your PCP or your surgeon or, sometimes, both. On occasion, surgeons and primary care physicians get into little turf wars over the post-surgical care of a patient. Since the last thing you want to have to do as you recover from surgery is to act as referee, get the lines of post-surgical authority straight before you have your operation. In that way, things are much more likely to run smoothly after your surgery.

Notes To The Chart

Being a physician has its advantages. One of them is knowing the best surgeons in the medical community. Patients of good primary care physicians have the same advantage, since good PCPs will refer their patients to the same surgeons that they would go to themselves. In fact, ask your PCP whether he or she or a member of his or her family has ever used the recommended surgeon for their personal medical needs. (Likewise, ask the surgeon you select which anesthesiologist he or she would use if the surgeon was going to have the same surgery you are planning.)

Finally, I cannot overemphasize the importance of storing your own blood in preparation for elective surgery. In fact, think twice and even three times before you agree to have surgery in a facility that does not offer this service. It really is important.

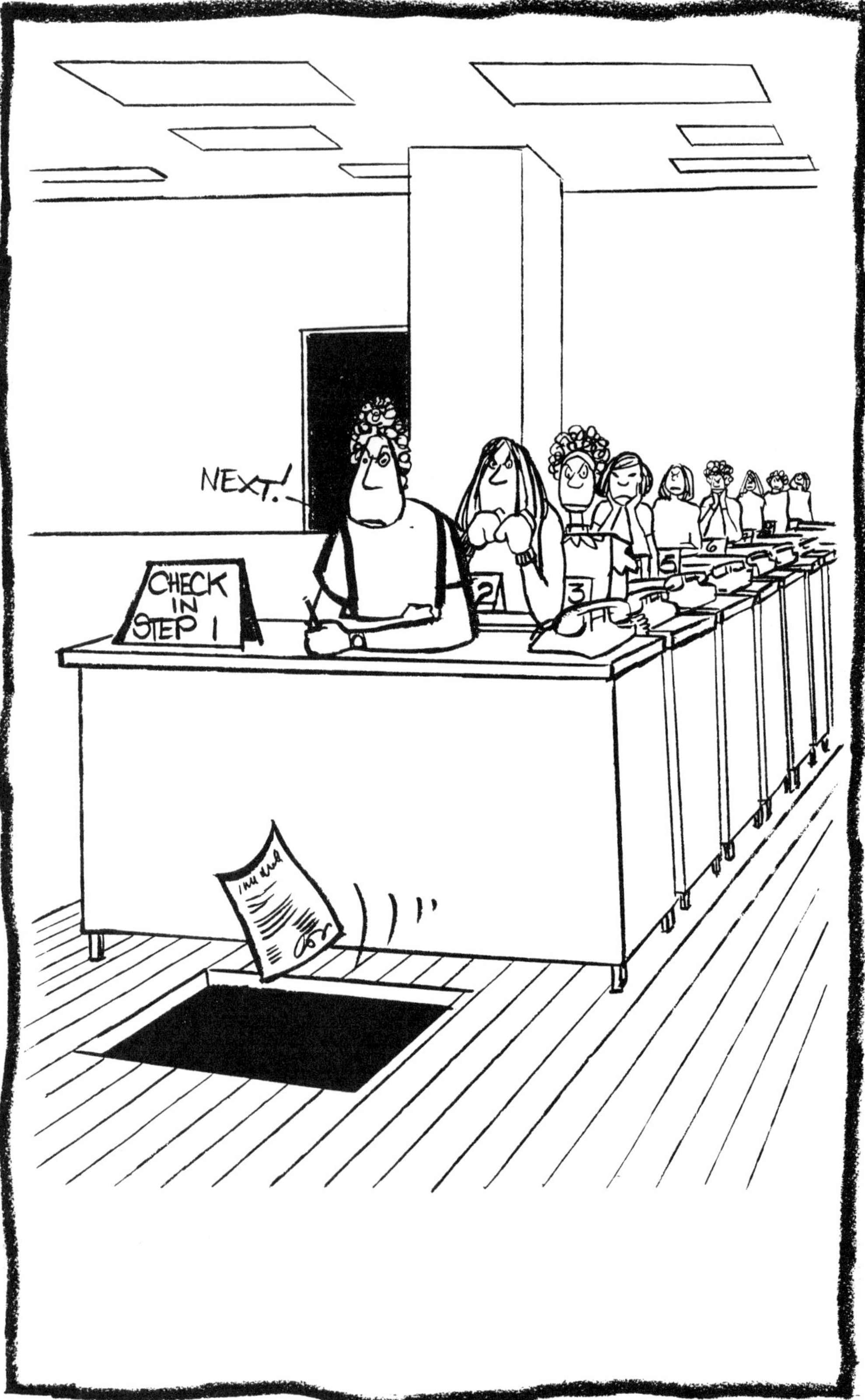
NEXT!
CHECK IN STEP 1

·9·

CHAPTER

Service With A Smile

• Hospitals and You •

When a patient checks into a hospital, the first thing he or she usually wants to do is check out, which is not surprising, since going to a hospital is not most people's idea of fun. Many seem to be cold, impersonal and depressing places, where the sick pay a small fortune to be treated (some claim with contempt), where the food makes airline fare seem like gourmet cooking and where the unpleasant scent of disinfectant never leaves the air. And so, it's no wonder that for many of us, when it comes to hospitals, "out of sight and out of mind" is the operating order of the day.

Since that is not a viable option for those who need hospitalization, the next best thing that patients can do for themselves (or which friends and relatives can do for their hospitalized loved ones), is make sure that their stay in the hospital is as humanized, comfortable and safe as possible. In other words, you can exercise patient power, even when you are flat on your back in the hold of a large hospital.

•Choosing The Right Hospital•

As you would expect, there are just hospitals and then again, there are *hospitals,* meaning that some institutions are far better than others. The trick for the medical consumer is to find that hospital which has just the right mix and balance of medical excellence and "hotel" comforts.

Medical excellence refers to the total ability of the hospital to adequately and competently provide the facilities, equipment and personnel for the optimum treatment of illness and injury. And not just the ability to treat the problem presented, but also the capacity to combat all of the common complications that can arise from the treatment or ailment. For example, if you are going to have open heart surgery, you will want the hospital you select to be capable of coping not only with the surgery itself, but with most of the potential problems that could arise.

The *hotel function* of a hospital is also of great importance to patients. Is the facility clean and comfortable? Are the rooms well lit and well decorated? Do the televisions work? Is the food good? In other words, is the facility managed in such a fashion that the patient will be made as comfortable as possible under the medical circumstances? After all, dreary, unclean, depressing surroundings are not exactly conducive to a prompt recovery.

It is your job as a patient, and the obligation of your doctor(s), to select the hospital that best combines the *medical* function and the *hotel* function to match your specific needs. Therefore, if you are going to have major surgery, the quality of the hospital intensive care unit will be far more important than the color of the curtains or the worn linoleum on the floor. On the other hand, a less serious matter may require less by way of medical back-up and more by way of the quality of the environment and length of visiting hours.

Here is a step-by-step approach to finding the right hospital for you:

Get Your Doctor's Recommendation

The person who will obviously have a great deal of say with regard to the choice of hospital is the doctor who admits you, be it your PCP, surgeon or sub-specialist. Usually your doctor will be limited in his or her recommendation to a hospital where he or she has staff privileges, although temporary privileges can sometimes be arranged. In any event, when your doctor recommends a hospital, make sure the doctor's primary reason for the choice is that it is *the best hospital to care for your particular problem.* Ask questions, such as "Why this hospital over others?" "What is your personal experience with this hospital that makes you believe that it is the right choice?" "Does the hospital have all that will be needed to care for me in the event of complications or will I require a transfer?" "Are the nurses well-trained and efficient?" "Does the hospital have a problem with hospital-acquired infection?" (Some critics charge that a number of hospitals are bad for your health due to the spread of staph and other infections to its patients.) In other words, make sure the recommendation is based on your medical needs and not solely upon the convenience or financial gain of the physician, such as an ownership interest in the facility.

Research the Hospital

There is a great deal of information available about your local hospitals, all just a phone call away. Here are some questions to ask your doctor or the hospital itself:

What is your JCAH rating? JCAH stands for the Joint Commission on Accreditation of Hospitals, an organization whose sole purpose is to encourage and enforce the attainment of uniformly high standards of institutional medical care. The commission periodically inspects each hospital, issues a report which describes the good, the bad and the ugly of each institution and informs the administrators both orally and in writing of the corrective action which must be taken for the hospital to comply with JCAH standards. The totality of the institution is covered by the status report, from the way the food is prepared, to the way medical charts are handled, to the ways in which the hospital makes staffing decisions, and everything in between—sort of the hospital equivalent of a complete physical.

Most importantly for the consumer, the JCAH also awards the hospitals it inspects an accreditation status, ranging from three years to probational (or, I suppose, no accreditation at all). If the accreditation is three years, then you know that the commission thought very highly of the institution. If it was probationary, you know that there were some serious problems. Of course, some problems may have little or no impact on patient care, but others clearly do, so if the hospital that you are thinking of going to has a low accreditation status, look closely into that institution to make sure that it is not a place that you would be advised to avoid. (By the way, if you are really ambitious, you can ask to read the report itself. But be prepared to spend some time at the task—the JCAH reports are usually twenty to thirty pages long.)

What complaints have been received by the State Health Department? If a consumer complains about a hospital to a State Health Department, generally that agency will conduct an investigation to see whether the complaint has merit and, if it does, corrective action will be taken by the administration. You, as a health care consumer, have the right to call the Health Department and ask, "What can you tell me about X Hospital?" You should be told what the JCAH status is and how the State Health Department views that facility. (Remember, the Health Department is a government agency which licenses and regulates the hospital, while the JCAH is a private accreditating organization. They may have differing views of the hospital, so it never hurts to find out the opinions of both.)

Ask your friends what their experience with the hospital has been. If you know someone who has been hospitalized in the hospital you are thinking of entering, ask whether the good times rolled or whether they were "dying" to get out. If there was a problem, find out the specifics and then discuss it with your doctor or the hospital so that you can head any potential trouble off at the pass.

May I inspect the hospital before I decide? If a doctor you trust recommends a hospital, the JCAH Accreditation is good, and the State Department of Health has had only minor complaints, you can be pretty well assured that the hospital you are interested in is not going to be bad for your health. Even so, there is one more thing you should do—call the administration office and ask for a tour. Walking through the facility will give you a very good idea about how the place *really* is (when no accreditation committee is expected). Look to see if the halls are clean. Do the nurses seem overworked or are they on top of the job? Are the personnel friendly or can you cut the hostility in the air with a knife? Is the hospital quiet? Does privacy seem to be respected? In other words, do the vibes make the hospital feel like a prince's palace or more like Dracula's castle?

Check Your Insurance Policy

As we've discussed, some insurance policies limit your choice of hospitals or require that you get prior approval before any non-emergency admission. If your policy places such restrictions upon you, make sure you comply with your contractual obligations before going in the hospital, unless, that is, you think bankruptcy would be a new and exciting experience.

• The Check-In •

When the decision is made to hospitalize, your doctor will contact the hospital and make a reservation for your care. At this time the hospital is told the purpose of your "visit" and the expected length of stay.

When you arrive at the hospital, overnight bag in hand, your first stop is the admitting area, where you will confront your first of many hurdles: the admissions clerk. The admitting process frequently makes patients feel worse than they already do. There is a rumor going around that as a prerequisite to employment, admissions clerks must take a special training course called Insensitivity Training, but in reality, they are not the reason for patient ill-ease. It's the process itself. Even though you may be ill or in pain, form after form will be thrust under your nose which you must sign before you can go to your room. You will be required to sign financial responsibility forms (if your insurance company doesn't pay, you will, and through the nose), an agreement to obey all hospital rules, a two-page description of patient rights and a generic general consent-to-treat form, to name just a few, and all in a span of ten minutes. If all of that doesn't make you feel a bit dehumanized, you will then be plopped into a wheelchair (even if you want to walk) and taken to your room.

Happily, there are some things you can do to make the admissions process a little easier to cope with:

Ask your doctor if you can sign all of the admission forms before you come to the hospital. Pre-admission is an excellent way to beat the dehumanized blues. If the forms are mailed to you so that you have ample time to read and digest what you are being asked to sign, the whole process will seem far less cold and mechanical. Besides, by filling out all of the forms ahead of time, you protect yourself by saving time and anxiety. This can be especially important if you are being admitted on the same day that you will be receiving surgery, a time when anxiety is the last thing you need to make your day.

Bring in a friend to handle the situation for you. Checking into a hospital is almost always stressful, not just because of the process itself but because of what is to follow. Frankly, most of us are just plain scared and thus we may not be operating on all cylinders. If "a friend in need is a friend indeed," then a friend *indeed* is one who will help a friend in need check into the hospital.

Make a point of being friendly. A smile is catching and friendliness can be downright contagious. Or, as the old saying goes, "What goes around comes around." So, if you're nice to the admissions clerk, you just might be given a little something extra, such as a room with a view.

Hint: One of the things that occurs in the admissions process is room assignment. Since most insurance companies will pay only for semi-private rooms, you are likely to have a roommate. Ask the clerk if you can be matched with another patient who is likely to have something in common with you. After all, the last thing anybody wants is to have to share a television with

---

a roommate who wants to watch rock videos twenty-four hours a day if your idea of fun is watching a rerun of "Polka Parade" (and vice versa).

Hint: The cost of a private room may be as low as twenty dollars per day over the price of a semi-private room. Considering the fact that many people crave privacy when hospitalized, the extra cost (which you are responsible for) may be well worth the price.

Also, ask your doctor if you can receive a private room for the cost of a semi-private room at your local hospital. With competition being what it is, if "business is slow," you just might get a bargain. Likewise, many hospitals will waive the Medicare deductible to get your business. Remember, it never hurts to ask your doctor to check into something for you.

Just because you escape the admissions clerk unscathed doesn't mean that you are going to receive immediate pampered service. The next part of check-in occurs when you go to your assigned room to meet the floor nurse who will finish the check-in process. Unfortunately, what sometimes happens is that you sit alone in your room for thirty or forty minutes waiting for some sign of human contact. (That's because someone may be having a major medical problem. Yes, triaging occurs, even here.)

Once the nurse *does* admit you, he or she proceeds with the nursing assessment, where you are asked everything from your bowel habits to how often you brush your teeth, all in a blunt fifteen-minute session. The intent of the nursing assessment is, of course, to better help the staff care for you; however, any ego that may have survived the admissions clerk intact is likely to be shredded along with the last vestiges of your privacy. By now, if you had any questions about the need for your hospitalization *before* admission, you will probably have no doubts about it any longer.

Hint: It is easy to feel two feet tall as you sit alone in a hospital room waiting to be told what to do. Bring a friend, or at least a good book, to make the process seem less lonely.

At some point, you will probably be asked to sign a specific medical consent form which details the specific treatment you are going to receive, along with most common potential complications. *Make sure your doctor is present, and not just a nurse, when you sign the consent form,* just in case you have any questions and to make sure that if you do, you get accurate answers. Remember, these forms are written by lawyers to reduce the chances that you will be able to sue later for malpractice, so you will not only have medical jargon to contend with, but "legalese." And so, be sure you fully understand what you are consenting to *before* you sign the form.

Hint: Sometimes these consent forms include "consents by omission," by which the failure to check off a box can constitute agreement to waive your legal rights. So be sure to read them carefully before signing.

• Your Tour Of Duty •

Many view their hospitalization as they would a tour of duty in the armed forces—it may be necessary, but boy, they can hardly wait to get out. However, unlike the military, your duty as a patient is not "to do or die," but to remain at the "cause" of your care, even when you are very weak or ill.

The best way to accomplish this feat of patient power is to recruit a friend or relative as your *patient advocate*, to help you care for your own comfort and, if necessary, medical needs. Your advocate will work on your behalf with the staff and your doctors to solve any problems that may arise with your care so that you don't have to settle for less than the best just because you're not strong enough to take care of yourself. Your choice for this advocate should be someone who is able to visit you frequently so that you have a chance to communicate about how you feel on a regular basis and so that the hospital personnel will know that there is someone on the outside who really cares about what happens to you.

The following is a list of the rights you have when you are hospitalized. Please note that in many states, these and other rights are established in law:

- You have the right to exercise your rights without regard to sex or cultural, economic, educational or religious background or the source of payment for your care.

- You have the right to be treated with respect and consideration by all hospital personnel.

- You have the right to know the name of the physician who is in charge of coordinating your care (the attending physician) and the names and professional relationships of other physicians who will consult with the attending physician.

- You have the right to receive *from the attending physician,* information about your illness, course of treatment and prospects for recovery, all in terms you can understand.

- You have the right to give your informed consent or to make an informed rejection and to otherwise actively participate in your own medical care.

- You have the right to privacy and the right to be told the reason that any individual might be present.

- You have the right to reasonable compliance with requests you make for service.

- You have the right to leave the hospital at any time, even against the advice of your physician (called discharge against medical advice).

- You have the right to continuity of care.

- You have the right to be advised if your care will be given in conjunction with a medical research project and to refuse to participate in the experimental care if you so desire.

- You have the right to be told about how best to continue your health care after discharge.

- You have the right to a clear, easy-to-understand, detailed bill, regardless of the source of payment, and to a detailed explanation thereof.

- You have the right to know the rules and hospital policies that apply to your conduct as a patient.

Knowing your rights is one thing, enforcing them is sometimes quite another. Here are some tips to help you make it through "the dark night" of your hospitalization.

If you are unhappy, speak to the staff member who is causing the problem (or have your patient advocate speak on your behalf). After all, there may be a good explanation why your call was answered late (such as a ward emergency) or why your food was cold.

If a particular nurse or orderly is consistently rude, slow or otherwise is not giving you the service you are paying a lot of money for, complain to the nursing supervisor. He or she should be able to solve your problem.

> **Hint:** If there is a nurse you really like or really don't like, make a point of asking the nursing supervisor to have that person assigned to you (or kept away). Your wish in that regard will generally be the supervisor's command.

Should the nursing supervisor be unable or unwilling to solve your problem, don't hesitate to go over his or her head right to administration. Most hospitals will give you the extension number of the administrative person whose job it is to resolve patient difficulties. Just pick up the phone and say, "I have a patient care problem. May I speak to someone as soon as possible?" That should get you results. If it doesn't, speak to your PCP or to another doctor. After all, if anyone has clout, they do, since they have the ability to steer their patients away from that particular institution.

Once you are out of the hospital and if you were unhappy with your care, you should write to any or all of the following:

- The administrator of the hospital
- The State Health Department
- The JCAH (875 N. Michigan Ave., Chicago, IL 60611)
- Your primary care physician

When you write the letter, be as precise as you can be about the problem and the personnel involved. List *facts* and *do not* get into name calling or an emotional diatribe. It will just serve to diminish your credibility. After all, you are trying to solve a problem for future patients, not just vent your spleen.

Also, if you write to complain (and even if you don't), let the hospital know what you *liked* about your treatment and care. Be sure to "name names." After all, people run hospitals, not machines, and a pat on the back or a shout of "Well done!" is as important to hospital personnel in their jobs as it is to you in yours.

• Teaching Hospitals •

Hospitals that are affiliated with medical schools, where clinical (hands-on) training is given, are generally called teaching hospitals. Teaching hospitals are different from other hospitals in many ways, some that benefit the patient and others that may not.

Patient care is often primarily handled by residents instead of board qualified or board certified physicians. Obviously, part of a teaching hospital's function is to teach, so it is not surprising that "students" will have direct and significant patient involvement. It is also important to understand that the residents (or interns) who work with patients in turn report to a board certified doctor who is usually called the "attending physician." Technically, the attending physician is the patient's doctor even though the resident may be the doctor (and I must emphasize that a resident *is* a doctor) who is usually seen. Thus, patients should make a point of meeting the attending physician if they have not done so and should use that board certified physician as a sounding board if they are unhappy with the care they are receiving from the resident. (For that matter they should also let the attending physician know when the resident has "done good.")

Hint: It is very important that patients who will be receiving long-term care at a teaching hospital ensure their continuity of care by getting to know the board-certified physician in charge of their treatment program, especially since residents will come and residents will go, but the attending physician is usually there to stay.

Hint: If you are admitted to a teaching hospital for surgery, make sure the surgeon *you have selected* will actually be performing the procedure rather than merely "supervising" a surgical resident that *you have not selected* as he or she does the job. If you are going to be used as teaching material, you have the right to know and approve of it in advance.

Teaching hospitals are frequently "tertiary care" centers and can thus provide more specialized care. The term "tertiary care," when associated with teaching hospitals, means that they are highly specialized centers which doctors rely upon when they, the sub-specialists and the local community hospitals have not been able to diagnose or adequately treat a medical problem. And so it is, then, that some teaching hospitals may have a highly specialized clinic which treats neurological disorders, while another may be known for its eye clinic and still another for its advanced care of coronary patients. When all else fails, your doctor may refer you to such a tertiary center in the hopes that residents and other doctors who focus on a very narrow scope of medical difficulty will be able to succeed where doctors with a more general approach may have failed.

You have far less privacy in a teaching hospital. While many of the tertiary care clinics that are found in teaching hospitals are outpatient facilities, there are times when patients are hospitalized in teaching hospitals. Those that are, whether for a specialized case or for a more common malady (after all, it is vital that doctors learn how to treat "normal illnesses" as well as unusual cases), will find that they have less privacy as their case is used as an example to residents, interns and others.

The care you receive should be among the best available. The payoff for that loss of privacy, however, is the fact that the teaching hospital may be on the cutting edge of medicine—a place where the attending physicians may be some of the best doctors in their respective fields and where the latest diagnostic tools will be available to help solve your medical problem. So what may be lost in comfort or privacy will be made up in medical excellence.

Teaching hospitals may be more expensive. Because of the expense associated with new technology, some hospitalizations that occur in teaching hospitals may be more expensive than those in a "regular" hospital (which also come in profit vs. nonprofit varieties). Thus, you may have a difficult time getting your insurance company or HMO to approve hospitalizations at such institutions unless you or your PCP or sub-specialist can convince them that the only way to give you adequate care is at such a facility.

Teaching hospitals may order more tests which can take longer to be processed. Remember, part of what happens in a teaching hospital is education. Thus, the residents who will be significantly involved in your care may order more tests than you might receive in another facility. Also, teaching hospitals tend to be very big places and so, service may be a little slow.

Hint: As with any other matter of your health care, you should be courteously assertive in your relations with the medical team at a teaching hospital. For example, you should know the names of all of the physicians who are charged with your care, each of their specialties and their specific role in the medical team that will be managing your case. You and your patient advocate should also know their respective telephone and/or beeper numbers. And whatever you do, just because you may be in a very famous institution of higher medical learning, don't be afraid to ask questions or to assert yourself.

• Home Free •

After your hospitalization is completed, your doctor will discharge you, at which time you will be "free" to go home. Once home, there is only one more thing you have to worry about regarding your hospitalization—the bill.

And what a bill it will be! Your basic room rate includes a bed, a nightstand, a television, three meals a day and basic nursing and housekeeping services. That's it. Everything else that you use during your stay, including aspirin (by the pill), bandages (by the gauze pad), and your use of all monitoring equipment or oxygen or other such necessities, will be billed as extras to the standard daily rate. Thus, your bill will, in all likelihood, be pages and pages in length and may be thousands and thousands in cost. (In all fairness, much of the individual packaging of items such as aspirin or laxatives are required by health codes and insurance companies which demand detailed billing statements.)

When you receive your bill, your first job is to not let its complexity or amount put you back into the hospital you were just released from. Your next job is to review it for errors, even though it will probably make your phone bill look like an elementary school math problem. According to Harvey Rosenfield, who works in affiliation with Ralph Nader in a consumer protection program called "The Bills Project," there are six areas in which hospitals are likely to overcharge their patients.

1. Indecipherable Bills: Some hospitals will itemize by computer number rather than listing the service or product being charged to your account. Under such circumstances it is impossible for you to know what the bill is for in the first place and whether or not you actually received the item being charged for. Also look out for the infamous "miscellaneous" charge, which takes your money but does not tell you what for. If either happens to you, ask for a bill that is detailed in fact as well as in theory.

2. Unitemized Bills: An unitemized bill might read "$14,000 for hospitalization from (date) to (date)." This is, of course, unacceptable. You wouldn't accept a receipt from a supermarket that reads "$127.65 for food purchased." Don't accept an equally ridiculous bill for far more money, over a far more momentous event in your life.

3. Excessive Charges: If you have been billed for an item in an amount that you think is in excess of its value, speak up. After all, it is one thing to pay one dollar for two aspirin, but six dollars!? (Yes, it has happened.)

4. Billing Fees: Some hospitals actually have the gall to charge you for preparing the bill! I mean they already charge for everything but the toilet paper! (To show you how bad it's getting, I was told by one hospital administrator that there is even a move afoot to charge patients for actual hours of nursing services rendered.) And since billing is a normal part of a hospital's business expenses, that fee should be covered in the basic room charge. Thus if you receive a bill with a charge for "processing fee" or "handling" or some other euphemism, make a fuss. In my opinion they have no business doing that.

5. Erroneous Charges: When you receive a bill that is twenty pages long, it is hard to spot mistakes. But they may be there, so look closely. If you were charged for an EKG that you never received, for example, speak up. If you are charged for medicine you don't remember receiving, complain. If you have been billed twice for the same service, get it erased. The cost of the services that were rendered are high enough, after all, without adding the expense of erroneous bills.

Hint: Pay special attention to the larger charges, since they are the ones that will really hurt. If you get overcharged $2.98 for a gauze pad it will be wrong, but it may cost you more in time lost than you will gain in money found to make a federal case out of a minor mistake. Remember, you are trying to convince a computer to change its data, and we all know how frustrating that can be.

Hint: Also watch out for the doctor who wasn't there. Some doctors claim to have checked in on their patients and billed them for the service when they were actually playing tennis.

---

6. Interest Charges on Mistakes: Talk about adding insult to injury, some hospitals will correct billing errors and fail to credit your account with any interest charged to your bill. Some people pay such improper interest charges out of pure frustration and a feeling of impotence. Don't be among them. It's your hospital's responsibility to give you an accurate bill, and it should not be allowed to get away with anything less.

If you have any questions about hospital or other billing abuses, or would like to share your tale of woe with someone who cares, contact The Bills Project, P.O. Box 1736, Santa Monica, CA 90406.

Once you have found a billing mistake, you should contact your insurance company and let them know. They'll work with the hospital to correct the error. In case they don't, you should also contact the hospital and let them know *in writing,* informing them of the mistakes you believe exist in your bill and demanding an *audit of your chart.* A chart audit involves a comparison of the medical bill with your actual medical chart. Mistakes that are caught are corrected, but they won't be caught if you don't ask. Here's a sample letter to use as a form:

Holy Cost Hospital
Attn: Patient Account Representative
3333 Golddigger Lane
Pickpocket, Wyoming 44444

Dear Sir or Madam:

I was hospitalized in your institution from May 5, (Year) until May 14, (Year). My attending physician was Dr. Laura Goodoctor (address and phone number), and I was also seen by a consultant, Dr. Peter Piper (address, etc.) over some pickled peppers that I had picked and which caused a serious allergic reaction.

I received my bill on May 28, and I found several errors that I would like you to correct. They are as follows:

5/5 $55 for EKG. I never received an EKG.

5/6 $28 for oxygen. While an oxygen unit was in my room, for which I have been billed, it was never used.

5/8 $18 for aspirin. I took two for a headache. I doubt whether they cost $9 apiece.

5/9 $111 for microscope. I don't understand that charge at all.

Please run a chart audit on my bill and advise in writing of the corrections you make. Also please reverse any interest charges on the incorrect items.

Thank you for your cooperation,

N.O. Patsy

N.O. Patsy
cc: Premium High Insurance Company

Hint: In any business dealings with a hospital, insurance company, or any other business entity for that matter, whether inside or outside the medical industry, always communicate in writing (whether as an original communication or a confirming letter over what was discussed orally) and keep copies for your records. That is called keeping a "paper trail" and it will allow you to reconstruct events should the need arise.

You should pay any part of the bill that is not in dispute since the hospital is clearly entitled to that money. However, you should not allow yourself to be bullied or coerced into paying a bill you do not owe. If you and your hospital cannot reach agreement, do not hesitate to make it prove its case in a court of law.

Notes To The Chart

The most frequent complaint I hear from my patients about their hospitalization has to do with delays in service. This usually involves the nurse's failure to run into the room the second the patient pushes the call buzzer. I make note of this because I rarely hear complaints about the response of nurses and other hospital personnel to medical emergencies or urgent care problems.

When we are ill, it is natural for us to get a bit grumpy and angry at what we perceive to be slow service, especially when we are paying hundreds of dollars per day for the "pleasure" of being hospitalized. However, please try to remember that the nurses, technicians and other hospital personnel are frequently overworked and underpaid. If any of us had to walk in a nurse's shoes for one working day, we would soon appreciate the dedication of these indispensable health care professionals.

All of that aside, if you are unhappy, follow the advice set forth in this chapter and speak up. Just try to do it politely.

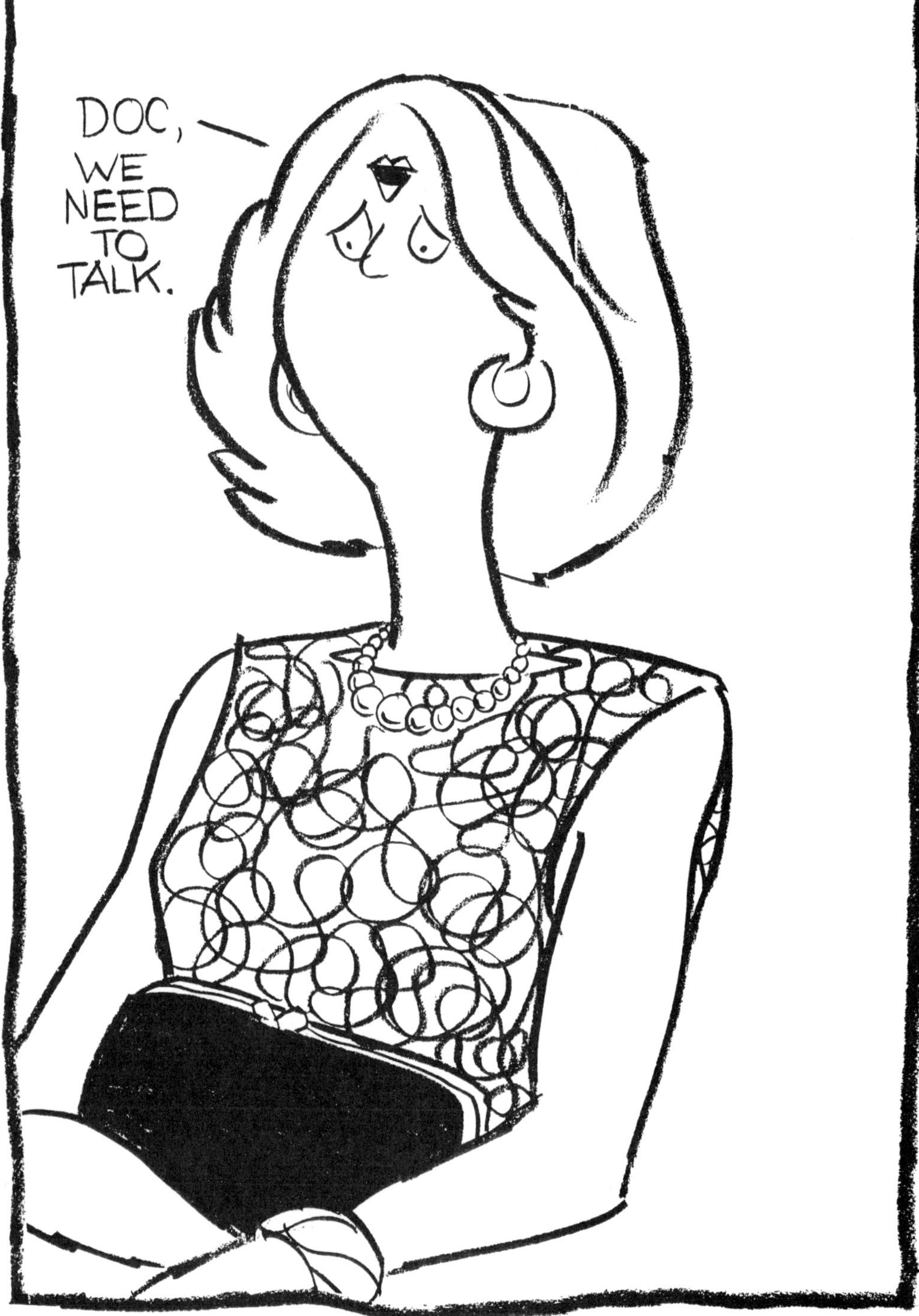
DOC,
WE
NEED
TO
TALK.

·10·

CHAPTER

The Fly In The Ointment

When Your Relationship · With Your Doctor · Turns Sour

I've got bad news and worse news. First the bad news. Sometimes individual doctors act in an unethical manner, do incompetent work and/or otherwise violate their responsibilities to their patients and their profession. Now, the worse news. Too often, little or nothing can be done about it.

The reasons for this weakness in the health care system are severalfold. For one thing, as we will discuss in greater detail, the only entities that can regulate a doctor's license to practice within each state are the individual State Licensing Boards. While these state agencies *do* have the power to revoke or suspend medical licenses, the areas of conduct which can result in such formal discipline are usually limited and the procedures involved are frequently very time consuming. Thus, while these state regulatory agencies do have teeth, the teeth are not very sharp.

As a result, much of the burden of policing unethical conduct falls upon doctors themselves. Yet they lack the power to force an unethical or incompetent doctor out of practice. Instead, they rely on peer pressure to bring about change.

The idea of professional self-regulation has been around for such a long time within the medical profession that it has become a tradition. Doctors, like lawyers, believe that the best way to deal with doctor/patient problems is to resolve them through the peer review process. The theory of peer review goes something like this: each doctor cares so much about what his or her colleagues think, that any unethical practice or incompetent performance will soon be corrected by the offending physician in order to avoid peer scorn and/or ostracism.

Unfortunately, what works in theory does not necessarily work in practice. Peer review can only be effective if the offending doctor does indeed care about how he or she is perceived by the medical community. Some simply do not. Secondly, in order to be subject to peer discipline, a doctor, with limited exceptions, must belong to a medical organization that has the power to apply sanctions against its members who refuse to change inappropriate behavior. If a doctor is not a member of a voluntary medical society, self-regulation becomes very difficult, since a nonmember is obviously not subject to the rules and regulations of a medical organization to which he or she does not belong. And since participation in these medical societies is purely voluntary, and because some doctors choose not to join any, or only join for outward appearances, there are physicians against whom little peer leverage can be applied (again, with some limited exceptions).

There are also problems of definition. What is unethical conduct? It seems that there are few objective standards upon which doctors and the care they render are judged. Each circumstance is viewed as unique, and phrases such as "beneath the standard of care" or "unprofessional conduct" are utilized to describe those activities or omissions that are deemed objectionable.

Finally, many doctors simply will not "rat" on other doctors even though, according to the Judicial Counsel of The American Medical Association, they are ethically obligated to "expose, without fear or favor, incompetent or corrupt, dishonest or unethical conduct on the part of members of the profession." Medical malpractice lawyers cynically call this reluctance to talk "the conspiracy of silence" (which doesn't really exist—there is no group of physicians who "conspire" to protect unethical colleagues). The tendency towards "silence," however, does exist and it doesn't involve just doctors who choose not to testify against their colleagues in a malpractice lawsuit (which many won't), but doctors who know about the "bad apples in the barrel" but who do little or nothing to take them out of circulation. (A problem that, in all fairness, the leaders of the medical community are working hard to overcome.)

Despite the difficulties that do exist, however, there are concrete steps that can and should be taken by a patient who believes that he or she has been treated improperly (professionally or otherwise) by his or her own doctor. *These steps require patient assertiveness.* Thus, if you are not prepared to "stand up and be counted," you'd better be prepared to take what you get, for without your active participation, nothing is likely to be done.

• Talk To Your Doctor •

The easiest and most effective way to solve problems that may arise between you and your own doctor is to deal with these difficulties directly with him or her in an open and honest manner. This "direct approach" works best if you and your doctor have established beforehand an open, honest and cordial relationship, in which both of you communicate with each other in a spirit of candor and mutual respect. In such an atmosphere are problems best solved; thus a *strong and effective patient/physician relationship is your first line of defense* against improper medical conduct.

Regardless of the strength or weakness of the tie that binds you to your doctor, if you do become disenchanted with your physician for any reason, by all means speak up. After all, your doctor is not going to be able to solve the problem if he or she does not know that a problem exists. Unfortunately, too many of us will complain to everybody *but* our doctor when we are unhappy, while pretending that nothing is wrong when we do see the physician with whom we are upset. In such ways do molehills become mountains.

But you don't just want to talk, you want to solve the problem. That means you have to more than just vent steam, you have to *communicate.* Here are some suggestions to help you do so:

Be Specific: It is not enough to tell your doctor that you are unhappy. You have to be able to express exactly *why* you are unhappy. Thus, be prepared to give specific examples of the conduct or omissions and the date(s) on which they occurred which lead you to believe you are receiving less than adequate care.

Avoid Emotionalism: To paraphrase Joe Friday of "Dragnet" fame, give your doctor the facts, Mr. or Ms. Patient, *just the facts.* It doesn't do you or your doctor any good if you express yourself behind a torrent of tears or if you engage in vitriolic name calling. Such conduct will only serve to cloud the issues and break the bonds of trust that have been forged between you.

Prepare for the Meeting: Many of us are in awe of doctors and do not feel adequate enough to confront them. If so, write down everything you want to discuss with your doctor before you meet with him or her "one-on-one." In this way, you will not "go blank" and will be able to put everything on the table that needs to be discussed. One word of advice: if you tend to get sweaty hands, use indelible ink.

Take Notes: Write down what your doctor tells you in response to your complaints. Remember, you are dealing in matters of great concern about which you may have little or no training. Thus, you will want to be able to digest what your doctor tells you and perhaps investigate it further, rather than make an immediate decision. Notes will help you remember what was said and will serve as a record of what transpired between you should there be further dispute.

Get a Second Opinion: If your disagreement with your doctor is over the quality of medical care or over your doctor's diagnosis or plan of treatment, by all means get a second opinion. As we have discussed, no doctor should ever be offended if you want a second opinion, and you will undoubtedly feel better if an independent opinion verifies the correctness of your doctor's approach. And if it doesn't, you and your doctor will have to sit down and decide how to proceed from there.

Write a Letter: Regardless of whether you and your doctor are able to resolve the problem, write a *confirming letter* to document the conversation or terms of your agreement so that there will be no questions later about what actually transpired between you. Such a letter will also serve as an objective reminder to your doctor about what was discussed so that he or she can take any action or implement any changes that may have been agreed upon. Here's an example of what I mean.

> Dr. I. N. Adequate
> 4444 Malpractice Pl.
> Babooshka, Wis. 99889
>
> Re: Our Conversation of October 5
>
> Dear Dr. Adequate:
> The purpose of this letter is to confirm the contents of our discussion of October 5, in which I brought the following to your attention:
> 1. I was unhappy with the length of time I have had to

wait in your waiting room before seeing you the last three times I have had an appointment. I understand that you cannot always control the medical circumstances which are presented to you and I appreciate your promise to make an extra effort to call me if you are running more than thirty minutes behind schedule.

2. I am glad you appreciate how frustrated I was when I felt rushed by you when you examined me on September 14. The pains I have been feeling in my arm were alarming me and when you didn't seem to take them seriously, I felt like my health was endangered. Thank you for explaining more fully why they do not concern you.

As you suggested, I have decided to get a second opinion. I have an appointment with Dr. Meredith Oversight, an internist in town. She will be in touch with you for copies of my records. Please let me know when they have been sent. I shall instruct her to contact you with her recommendations and conclusions so that we can decide together how I should proceed.

Thank you for agreeing to discuss my concerns with me. I really do appreciate your medical skills and value our relationship.

Sincerely,

Mary Goodpatient

Mary Goodpatient

If you take the time to resolve the difficulties with your doctor in an open and non-accusatory fashion, the great majority of problems will be resolved then and there. However, if talk doesn't do the trick, it's time to take serious action and find a new doctor.

• Getting A New Doctor •

As we have discussed, doctors in private practice are professionals, but they are also business persons who seek the good life through their careers in medicine. As the number of doctors in the country has increased, competition within the business of practicing medicine has intensified, making each patient more important to his or her doctor's financial health. Therefore, one of the most effective ways to express your displeasure with a doctor "who has done you wrong" is to take your business elsewhere.

Only you can decide when the time has come to find a new doctor. Maybe you aren't happy with the results of the medical treatment you have been given or perhaps you don't feel like your doctor treats you with the respect and courtesy you deserve. But whatever the cause, if the bonds of trust and confidence so important to the physician/patient relationship have been broken beyond repair, the time has come to find new medical talent.

If you do decide to make a change in doctors remember the following:

Maintain Continuity of Care: Never fire your old doctor until you have found another one to take his or her place, especially if you are suffering from an illness or condition which requires ongoing care. Otherwise you may find yourself sitting for hours waiting in an emergency room for treatment that might otherwise be a phone call away.

Choose Well: Changing doctors is a traumatic experience under the best of circumstances, somewhat akin to getting a divorce. So do yourself a favor and choose your next doctor carefully. In that way, you won't have to spend the time, energy and emotion going through the whole process all over again.

Have Your Medical Records Forwarded: Your new doctor will need copies of your medical records from your old doctor, so don't be afraid to give him or her the old doctor's name and phone number, or ask your previous doctor to forward them yourself. Also, don't become paranoid if your new doctor decides to discuss your condition with your old doctor by thinking that the old doctor will try to poison the new doctor against you. It definitely should not be done.

Let Your Old Doctor Know That He Or She Is Off The Case: Being someone's doctor is a heavy responsibility that carries with it many duties to perform. So be fair. Once you have found a new doctor, let your old one know that his or her services are no longer required. It's the only decent thing to do.

Tell Your Old Doctor Why You Left: Sometimes doctors lose patients and they don't know why. Perhaps it's a staff member or maybe it's the doctor's attitude toward patients. Whatever it was for you, let the doctor know. In that way other patients may be spared the trouble you experienced which inspired you to make the change.

Despite the pessimistic introduction to this chapter, you should not ignore unethical or improper conduct (as opposed to non-ethical matters such as personality differences) which you have experienced at the hands of your doctor. Instead, if you are a victim of improper medical conduct, definitely report it to the proper authorities. It's the only way the system has any chance of working.

To Your State Licensing Board

Each state has a Licensing Board which has the responsibility of licensing doctors to practice within the state and which is charged with disciplining doctors who practice their duties in an unprofessional manner. While the laws and procedures vary from state to state, the system, which is a bureaucrat's dream, generally works as follows: A doctor is reported by a patient, another physician or some other interested party to the state board. An initial determination is then made as to whether the complaint falls within the board's jurisdiction. In order for the state to be able to take disciplinary action, the offense will generally be:

- Incompetence
- Gross negligence (not making a mistake, but an extreme deviation in care)
- Repeated negligent acts
- Falsifying medical reports
- Fraudulent medical claims, i.e., as against Medicare
- Mental or physical illness which substantially impairs the ability of the physician to practice medicine safely
- Abuse of drugs or alcohol
- Prescribing dangerous drugs without a medical exam
- Intoxication while attending a patient
- Other matters less directly related to patient care, such as conviction of crime

If the board investigator does not feel the matter comes within the state's jurisdiction, it will be referred to the doctor's local medical association for peer action. If it does come within the board's lawful jurisdiction, an investigation is undertaken, culminating (eventually) in a written report advocating a dismissal or recommending an action be filed seeking to discipline the doctor under investigation.

The matter is referred to the proper state authority, usually the attorney general's office, which reviews the file, investigates the case some more and, if it is deemed appropriate, files a complaint.

An administrative hearing is then held, which is akin to a full-fledged trial, in which the state tries to prove the doctor acted improperly and the doctor defends him- or herself.

If the administrative judge recommends discipline, the state licensing board reviews the file, the judge's conclusions of fact and law and makes an order for discipline, which can range from license revocation to private censure.

If the doctor doesn't like the board's action, he or she can appeal the decision by suing the board, claiming that the decision to discipline was improperly reached or was inappropriate to the violation.

The state courts then get into the action and the matter can go right up the appeals court ladder until eventually the matter is finally resolved.

As you can see, the discipline process is a long and arduous one, filled with legal protections for the doctor to make sure that his or her license is not revoked or suspended without due process of law. On the other hand, justice delayed is justice denied, and it is no wonder that many feel inadequately protected by these formal disciplinary proceedings.

Note:
Each state handles its medical disciplinary proceedings differently. If you want details of the procedures or the grounds for discipline in your respective state, contact your state licensing board at the address and phone number listed in the supplement.

Peer Review

Medical Societies: Consumer complaints that are of insufficient seriousness to justify state discipline are handled by national medical associations such as the AMA, or local societies such as a state or county organization, assuming, that is, that the offending doctor is a member. Each association handles complaints against its members differently, but generally the process works something like this: When a complaint is received, a volunteer physician who is a member of the association's ethics committee will contact the complaining party and the accused physician to determine whether formal action needs to be taken. An attempt will also be made to mediate the differences between the doctor and patient to see whether the problem can be solved in that manner so that no formal action is required. If this effort fails and if the physician is found to be at fault, he or she will receive a letter from the association asking that the inappropriate behavior be corrected. In cases of repeated violations or serious ethical breaches, discipline may be imposed, ranging from public censure to the removal of the offending doctor from the referral list, or expulsion from the organization.

Matters that are dealt with in local associations include fee disputes, misdiagnosis caused by improper examining techniques, improper communication with a patient, and any other matter of concern to a patient that falls beneath the threshold of "unprofessional conduct" which would require state action.

Hint: If a doctor is not a member of a medical society, there is very little peer review that can take place, leaving the patient totally without protection, except for state action, which is difficult to obtain and which takes a very long time to complete. Consequently, it is a good idea to choose a doctor for yourself who maintains an active membership in a local medical society. Otherwise you may have no one to turn to if you have a problem with the doctor.

Hospitals: Hospitals are able to exercise a certain amount of control over the medical care rendered by physicians because of their power to revoke staff privileges. A doctor who has been removed from a staff will no longer be able to treat patients in that hospital, which can restrict the doctor's practice and thus reduce his or her income. A doctor removed from the staff will also be removed from the hospital's referral list, thereby reducing the flow of new patients. So, if you have been treated by a physician who has given you improper medical care, especially if it occurred in the hospital, write a letter to the hospital administrator detailing your complaints. That will definitely get your doctor's attention, and more importantly, serve as an incentive for the doctor to change his or her ways.

Medical Groups, Insurance Companies or HMOs: Many doctors practice these days as part of a medical group, such as a PPO or IPA (see Chapter 5), or otherwise have a special relationship with a medical insurance company. As with hospitals, the displeasure of these entities or groups can have a severe impact on the doctor's bank account. This gives you leverage. Thus, if you are unhappy with a doctor you have seen who is connected with a health insurance group, write a little letter to the plan administrator detailing your complaints. You might be surprised at how quickly the doctor changes his or her tune.

• Sue Your Doctor •

It's time to talk about the "M" word— *malpractice.* If there is one thing that makes doctors go rabid, it is malpractice. If there is one area of the law that strikes fear and loathing into an insurance executive's heart, it is malpractice. If there is one "consumer sword" which has forced the medical field to improve its art, it is malpractice. But if there is one concept that medical consumers really know little or nothing about, you guessed it, it is malpractice.

The Nature Of The Beast

Medical malpractice occurs when a physician (or hospital or other health care professional) renders negligent medical care to the patient, resulting in damages. The following elements must be proved in order to win a malpractice lawsuit:

1. The care rendered by the physician was *beneath the standard of care* within the doctor's medical community. That doesn't mean the patient didn't get better or even that the wrong course of treatment was selected; it means that the doctor did not exercise the degree of knowledge and medical skill that a "reasonable physician" under the same circumstances would have exercised. Sounds subjective? It is. How do you prove that the treatment fell beneath the standard of care? Testimony by other doctors. How easy is it to get that testimony? Not very.

2. The patient must have *suffered damages* which were *caused* by the delivery of *substandard medical care.* That is, it is not enough to prove that the doctor was negligent. It must also be proved that the patient suffered damages to health or pocketbook because of the negligent care. This isn't always easy. Many doctors defend malpractice cases by alleging that the negligence did not change the ultimate outcome in a significant way.

For example, assume that a doctor doesn't catch an advanced case of lung cancer for one month beyond the time a reasonable doctor would have. The cancer victim dies. It is unlikely that the family would be able to win a lawsuit for malpractice because of the almost impossible burden of proving that the deceased patient would have lived longer or experienced significantly less pain and suffering. On the other hand, a doctor who mistakenly takes out the wrong kidney will have a much more difficult time defending a malpractice suit, since it will be far easier to prove substandard care and resulting damages to the patient's health and welfare.

It is almost impossible to list all of the negligent acts which have been found to be malpractice since each case must, by definition, be judged on its own merits. For example, a misdiagnosis may or may not be malpractice. Likewise, failure to give informed consent will only be judged malpractice if it can be shown that:

1. The patient *would not have consented* to the treatment if he or she had been informed of the risks and

2. The treatment, as delivered, *caused actual damages.* Failure to refer to a specialist cannot be adjudicated as malpractice unless the doctor knew or should have known that he or she did not have the knowledge or skill to treat the patient.

Now, add to all of that hedging and equivocating the fact that each state has different laws regarding malpractice, and you can begin to see just how confusing the field of malpractice can be.

What To Do If You Are A Malpractice Victim

Confusing or not, if you believe you have suffered significant damage to your health, well-being or pocketbook at the hands of a negligent doctor, you must be ready to take action. Here are some suggestions on what to do.

• **Obtain your medical records:** This is essential because there is no way for a lawyer or another doctor to evaluate the treatment you received unless they have your records to review. Plus, a few doctors and hospitals have been known to change records to make themselves look better (the motion picture *The Verdict* was not altogether fanciful). And so you will want accurate records before the lawsuit explodes in your doctor's face.

• **Consult another doctor:** Remember, just because everything didn't turn out exactly the way you and your doctor wanted doesn't mean that malpractice was committed. Therefore, if you suspect something may be wrong, ask another doctor—not to be a witness, but for an honest appraisal of your condition.

• **See a lawyer:** I know that sounds like suggesting that you jump into shark-infested waters with a bleeding hand, but there is just no way you are going to be able to deal with legal intricacies or insurance company maneuvers without a good lawyer by your side (with emphasis on the word *good*). Besides, there is no way you are going to know if you really have a case unless you get the opinion of a medical malpractice lawyer. When it comes to selecting a lawyer, consider the following:

Experience: Make sure the lawyer is experienced in the field of medical malpractice. As you have seen, the field is complicated and frustrating and requires a great deal of medical knowledge and expertise on the part of the lawyer. Also, an experienced malpractice lawyer is going to have access to medical experts willing to testify on your behalf, which other lawyers may not have. Obviously, a divorce lawyer is just not going to cut it.

Hint: When interviewing a prospective lawyer be sure to ask how many malpractice cases he or she has handled and how many have been taken to trial. This is because insurance companies generally know the lawyers willing to take a case to trial and those that are eager to settle.

Expense: Most medical malpractice matters are paid for by the contingency fee where the lawyer keeps a defined percentage of the money collected in the case. If no money is collected, no fee is owed.

However, this is not a risk-free proposition for clients. There is something called "costs" in any lawsuit, which are the expenses which must be paid to others who help carry forward the lawsuit. In a medical malpractice suit, you will have to pay doctors, court reporters for deposition expenses, photocopying companies, court clerks and many others to help prove your case. These costs can run into the thousands of dollars, and the client is responsible, regardless of whether the case is won or lost.

Hint: Ask your lawyer if he or she will "advance" costs on your behalf and then accept repayment out of the lawsuit proceeds. Many will, which will keep you from having to choose between your lawsuit and your mortgage payment.

Disclosure: Lawsuits are time-consuming, emotionally draining and difficult endeavors at best, and you must be prepared for what is to come if you are going to be able to have any semblance of a normal life. So be sure to ask the lawyer *what* is going to be happening step-by-step and *when* before you proceed. You may just decide that it isn't worth the agony to file the lawsuit.

Hint: Many states have reacted to the malpractice insurance crisis and have given in to doctor and insurance company pressure by making it very difficult for malpractice victims to obtain competent legal representation. This is usually done by limiting the amount of contingency fees lawyers can charge and by limiting the amount of damages for pain and suffering that can be awarded (not out-of-pocket money paid for the pain and suffering created by the malpractice!). And yet, nothing is done to restrict what defense lawyers can do to defend against malpractice suits. Thus don't be surprised if you find it difficult to obtain a lawyer in smaller cases, leaving you in a situation where you have suffered a wrong without a remedy.

Note:
For more details on how to hire and work with a lawyer, please refer to THE LAWYER BOOK. *(Price Stern Sloan, 1986, by the author.)*

• **Live your life.** A lot of people tend to put their lives on hold when they get involved with a personal injury lawsuit (which is what a malpractice case is). This is a mistake. You only live once and no lawsuit is worth living less than the best you can under the circumstances.

NOTES TO THE CHART

The great majority of physicians are competent, dedicated, ethical individuals who give their patients quality medical care. But people are not machines and it is not uncommon for individual patients to have illnesses that are not "textbook" cases. If every patient had the same symptoms and test results for each disease, computers would replace doctors. But they don't, so doctors will always be with us.

The malpractice insurance crisis has shaken the very foundations of the American medical system, which I consider to be the finest in the world. I don't mean to be theatrical, but it is becoming very difficult to practice medicine in an atmosphere that generates mistrust between doctor and patient. And even though the great majority of malpractice cases that go to trial are resolved in favor of the doctor, the cost in stress and money (including escalating insurance rates) can be very high indeed. These costs are eventually borne by the patient since they are ultimately recovered in higher fees. The threat of malpractice also induces doctors to practice "defensive medicine" through ordering more tests and consulting more sub-specialists, which the patient also pays for.

The best way to deal with improper medical care is, truly, to avoid it in the first place. Choose your doctors well and maintain an active participation in your own health care. Such a partnership builds mutual trust and confidence and will go a long way toward keeping you out of the malpractice lawyer's office and you and your doctor out of court.

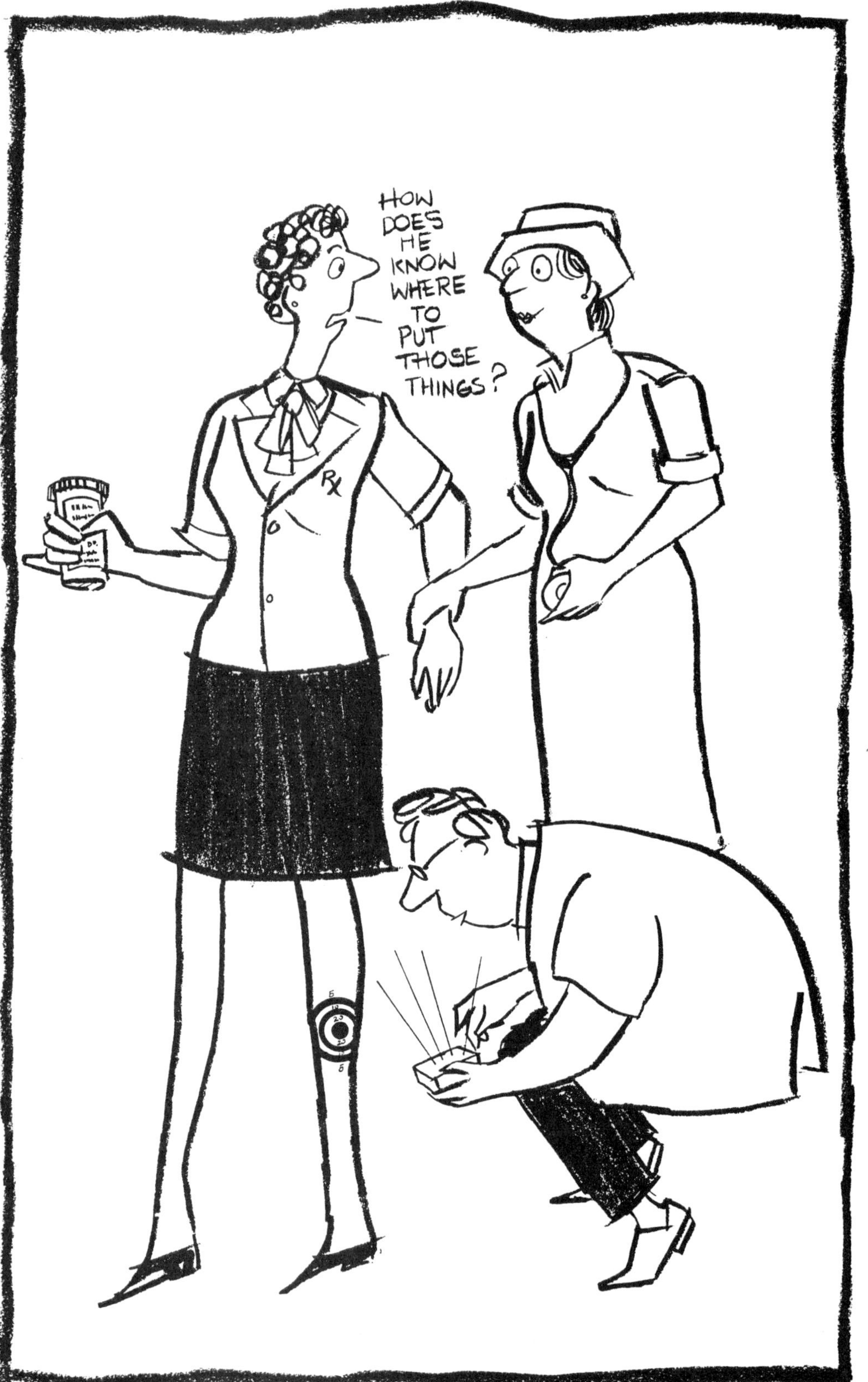
HOW DOES HE KNOW WHERE TO PUT THOSE THINGS?

·11·

CHAPTER

They Also Serve Who Are Not M.D.s

The Role of Other Health Care Professionals

This book has primarily concerned itself with the doctor/patient relationship and the workings of the health care delivery system as it relates to traditional medical care. That does not mean, however, that doctors are the "be all and end all." Far from it. For, while doctors may be the "stars" of modern medicine, there are many other professionals who rightfully deserve to take their place in the spotlight as co-stars and featured players in the delivery of health care to us all.

NOTE: Much of this book has equal application to your interaction with the professionals we are about to discuss as it does to M.D.s. That is, you as a patient have just as much right to participate in your own health care with a chiropractor as you do with an internist, and you have equal obligations to both. In other words, if you are the patient of an osteopath, feel free to call this book *The Osteopath Book*, or if you are being treated by a chiropractor, I won't sue if you call it *The Chiropractor Book* (just don't tell my agent).

Chiropractors

Historically, doctors have disliked chiropractors—or at least, the American Medical Association has. For years the "Chiro Wars" have raged, sometimes in the courts, sometimes in the discussion of public affairs, but usually hot and heavy over the proper role, if any, of chiropractors in the delivery of health care.

Those battles still rage to some extent, but the existence of chiropractors as legitimate members of the health care field is no longer in doubt. In fact, chiropractors are licensed in all fifty states, while health insurance and Medicare pay for chiropractic treatment and, most importantly, millions of Americans swear by the profession.

What Chiropractors Do

The approach of a chiropractor is definitely different from that of a medical doctor's. Chiropractors believe that good health depends to a large degree upon a normally functioning and well-balanced nervous system. Balance, according to this view, depends upon the correct alignment of the vertebrae and related nerve centers. If the nervous system is not balanced, the nerve roots of the spine become irritated, which in turn upsets the balance of the body, leading to certain bodily malfunctions which leave the whole organism vulnerable to disease. Thus, great emphasis is placed upon keeping the spine properly "aligned."

Chiropractors believe in preventive care and recommend that patients see them on a regular basis to have their spines examined so that deviations from the norm can be caught before they cause problems either in the back or elsewhere in the body. The frequency of such preventive examinations should be discussed with your chiropractor.

Chiropractors also have great faith in the body's innate ability to heal itself, and so promote a holistic approach to health care that does not use drugs or surgery to effect cures. The principal weapon in the chiropractor's healing arsenal is the spinal *adjustment* where deviations from normal spinal alignment are corrected, allowing the energy which flows through the nervous system to move normally through the body. This, in turn, allows the body to cure itself. Chiropractors also use other therapies (which are also utilized by physical therapists and others) such as *ultrasound* (use of high-frequency sound to reduce muscle spasms and increase nerve flow) and *diathermy* (a high-frequency current used to produce deep heat) as well as other therapies, ranging from nutritional guidance to traction.

Hint: If you go to a chiropractor, be sure that you understand what the doctor intends to do and *why,* along with the possible side effects, the alternatives and the hoped for benefits, before consenting to treatment, just as you would (or should) with a physician.

More About Chiropractors

They are licensed: Chiropractors are licensed in all fifty states. Their degree is a D.C. (Doctor of Chiropractic), which can be obtained after extensive training requiring a minimum of two years of college work and four years of chiropractic college followed by a clinical internship.

They can diagnose: Chiropractors are allowed to give physical exams and can order diagnostic tests such as blood tests or x-rays. Their physical exam is very similar to the one administered by a physician (see Chapter 6), with the addition of a physical evaluation of the structure and function of the spine. (Chiropractors in general place a much greater emphasis on x-rays of the spine than do M.D.s.) Chiropractors are permitted to diagnose all ailments. However, if the diagnosis is one which requires treatment which chiropractors cannot give, the patient *must* be referred to a physician.

Hint: Chiropractors increasingly have doctors to whom they will refer patients for nonchiropractic care. If your chiropractor tells you that you do indeed need a doctor, be just as careful in your selection of the physician as you would otherwise be (see Chapter 2). In other words, your chiropractor's referral should be treated as any other professional referral, no more and no less.

They can treat: While most people associate chiropractic care with the treatment of back and neck pain, chiropractors are permitted to treat a far wider scope of ailments including nonallergic asthmas, spastic colon and headaches. The principal method of treatment is again the spinal adjustment, or the manipulation of other areas of the musculoskeletal system.

But chiropractors cannot prescribe any medication that is not obtainable off the shelves.

They cannot conduct "invasive procedures": If you as a patient need an injection, a blood test, transfusion or surgery, your chiropractor will not be the person to perform the procedure, since they are not permitted to undertake any treatment or test which breaks the skin.

Also, they cannot treat all ailments: While there are some ailments that chiropractors can treat in addition to back and neck pain, there are many more than they cannot treat, including (but not limited to): cancer, infections, internal injuries, lacerations and cuts, fractures of bones and chronic ailments such as high blood pressure or diabetes.

Hint: If you have a malady for which you seek treatment from a chiropractor, make sure it comes within the range of illnesses which he or she is permitted to treat. If in doubt, consult a physician.

Chiropractors cannot hospitalize: With very rare exceptions, chiropractors do not have staff privileges at hospitals and thus cannot hospitalize patients or treat them if they are, as the British say, "in hospital."

Hint: While many doctors refuse to work with or accept the validity of chiropractic care, some have "loosened up" and have developed professional relationships with D.C.s, working with chiropractors to provide integrated patient care.

For more information on chiropractors, contact the American Chiropractic Association, 1701 Clarendon Blvd., Arlington, VA 22209, or your state or local chiropractic society.

• Osteopaths •

An osteopath is an interesting cross between an M.D. and a chiropractor. On the one hand, they are full-fledged physicians who can do virtually everything that a medical doctor can do, including surgery and prescribing. Yet on the other hand, they believe in and engage in spinal and other "manipulations" in a manner similar to chiropractors.

Osteopaths view the body as a single, individual organism where each and every body part relies on every other part to function properly. In other words, the body is completely interdependent and a malfunction of one part affects every other part; and therefore, if one part of the body is sick, the entire body is sick.

Osteopaths, like chiropractors, place great emphasis on the body's ability to heal itself and upon the importance of the nervous system in maintaining body health. And, while osteopaths place greater emphasis on the circulatory system than chiropractors do, both agree that a disturbance in the circulatory or nervous system affects the proper functioning of the body as a whole.

Osteopaths offer the following medical services:

Diagnosis: D.O.s (Doctors of Osteopathy) use all of the medically accepted tools of diagnosis including history, examination and testing. In addition, they use their hands to detect "structural" abnormalities of the spine or other parts of the skeletomuscular system in an attempt to detect defects which could cause disease or other body malfunctions.

Prevention: Like chiropractors and, increasingly, like M.D.s, osteopaths place great emphasis on preventive care, with nutritional guidance and exercise programs topping the list of preventive care.

Traditional medical care: Osteopaths place great emphasis on "natural healing," but do not shrink from engaging in the same medical and surgical procedures as medical doctors when they believe such treatments are warranted. And so, unlike chiropractors, D.O.s can engage in invasive procedures, prescribe medications and become members of hospital staffs. There are more than 200 "osteopathic hospitals" around the country which accept the theories of osteopathic care.

Manipulative treatments: Osteopaths use manipulations to correct structural problems, improve poor posture and otherwise improve the "flow" of the nervous and circulatory systems. Unlike chiropractors, however, D.O.s usually use manipulation in concert with other forms of medical care.

Here are some other interesting facts about osteopathic medicine.

• Osteopaths must take four years of college, four years of osteopathic training at an osteopathic college and one year of internship to receive a state license as a Doctor of Osteopathy.

• Some osteopaths choose to specialize. If they do, they must take a residency program of between two and six years, depending on the specialty selected.

• Osteopaths have their own state licensing boards and hospital accreditation procedures which are independent of the JCAH.

• Most osteopaths practice general or primary care.

• Osteopaths are most often found in smaller communities, and are frequently the only physicians available in such communities.

• The largest concentration of osteopaths can be found in the states of Michigan, Pennsylvania, Ohio, New Jersey, Florida, Texas, Missouri and Oklahoma.

• There are over 20,000 osteopaths in the United States, who treat 25 million Americans each year.

• Health insurance and Medicare will pay for osteopathic care.

For more information on osteopathic medicine, contact the American Osteopathic Association, 212 East Ohio St., Chicago, IL 60611.

Podiatrists

Podiatrists are not M.D.s as many think, but are a health care profession unto themselves, with their own education and licensing requirements.

Podiatrists are medical specialists of the feet, toes, ankles and tendons that run into the foot. Podiatrists are able to perform surgery and most commonly treat bunions, hammertoes, warts, ingrown toenails, corns, calluses and heel pain. Due to the physical fitness craze, podiatrists are increasingly treating stress-related foot problems as well as a greater number of fractures and sprains.

Podiatrists are not permitted to amputate and may only administer local anesthesia. If the foot problem is found to be a symptom of a disease such as diabetes, rather than the malady itself, a podiatrist must refer the patient to a qualified physician for treatment of the underlying condition. Podiatrists may, however, prescribe medications which are consistent with foot care, such as antibiotics or pain pills.

To become a podiatrist, a student generally must obtain a bachelor's degree and attend four years of podiatric medical school. Most states also require a one-year residency as well as passing written and oral exams as prerequisites for licensing.

Nurses

The key word when it comes to nurses is the word *"under,"* as in *under*paid, *under*appreciated and too frequently, mis*under*stood. Underpaid because the money they receive does not equal the responsibility they are given. Underappreciated because they are frequently taken for granted by both doctors and patients; and misunderstood because few truly appreciate the depth of a nurse's training and how much he or she really does to promote a patient's health.

Then what *do* they do, you ask? You name it. They conduct physicals. They engage in medical research. They direct paramedics as they rush to hospitals with a critically ill or injured patient. They work for insurance companies reviewing the appropriateness of care. They manage chronic illness, administer anesthesia and deliver babies. And, of course, they perform their traditional function of caring for the ill in hospitals. In fact, one of the few things they do not do is surgery, and even then, some states permit them to assist.

Of course, not all nurses engage in all areas of practice. Nurses are becoming almost as specialized as doctors. Here's a brief rundown of some of the different areas of nurse "emphasis":

Nurse Practitioner: Nurse practitioners (NPs) generally have a master's degree level of education and are permitted to give physical exams, order and interpret tests and manage common illnesses. In some states they are even permitted to prescribe medications. NPs generally manage "well health" care, and can be found working for HMOs, outpatient clinics and as the assistant of a private practice physician. Nurse practitioners also "sub-specialize" in areas such as pediatrics, cardiology and geriatric care (care for the elderly).

Certified Nurse Midwife: These practitioners deliver babies and meet the gynecological needs of healthy women.

Clinical Nurse Specialist: These highly educated practitioners are usually in charge of educating hospital nursing personnel, writing "protocols" of care and consulting with nurses about handling patients with difficult problems. They also engage in clinical research.

Registered Nurses: When most people think of nurses, they think of the hard-working R.N., who can be found in hospitals, in doctors' offices, visiting nurses associations and, in fact, everywhere nursing services are needed. R.N.s do so much, including:

- Carrying out the medical regimen (such as giving pills, administering injections, starting IVs, changing dressings, etc.)

- Assisting the patient's emotional adjustment to his or her malady and/or hospitalization

- Helping families cope with the illness of loved ones

- Educating patients and families in the methods of self-care

- Monitoring a patient's physical status, which these days frequently means working with computers and very sophisticated machinery, as well as the expected monitoring of vital signs and progress of healing

- Alerting doctors to problems the patient is experiencing

- Serving as a fail-safe against incompetent, unethical or illegal doctor care (i.e., spotting mistakes, or nagging a doctor to give appropriate tests, etc.)

- Making sure the patient and his or her environment is kept clean, comfortable, quiet and as private as is practicable

- Coordinating the "medical team," such as a social worker, dietician or chaplain when patient care problems have been discovered

---

Hint: If you or a loved one are hospitalized, make a point of establishing a good relationship with the nursing staff. Be friendly and assertive regarding the quality of care, but also be understanding. Remember, your nurse has a lot of patients to care for. Also, family members should make a point of being present. Family visits go a long way toward ensuring quality of care.

Licensed Vocational Nurses: LVNs are the foot soldiers of health care. In other words, they perform the dirtiest tasks and receive the least credit of the professionals who work in health care. I mean, think about how lousy life could quickly become without bedpan service. Of course, LVNs do much more than that—they are the task-oriented workers who perform varied chores, usually under the direction of R.N.s or other nurses with a higher degree of training.

A Note Regarding Home Nursing Care:

Due to the great emphasis being placed on cutting the costs of medical care, many patients are now sent home from hospitals before they once were, or are not hospitalized at all. Thus, private duty nursing services are becoming more important than ever before.

Private duty nursing is designed to provide the same nursing services at a patient's home that would be provided if the patient were hospitalized. Emphasis is also placed on patient and family education since the nurse is usually not available more than a few hours per day or a few days per week. Homemaker services can also be obtained where appropriate. Such services are usually obtained by contracting with a Visiting Nursing Association in conjunction with a physician's order for such care.

• Midwives •

For centuries, women have been having babies in the same old-fashioned way. Only in relatively recent times has childbirth been treated more as an illness than a natural act, requiring hospitals, anesthesia and a great deal of medical fuss and bother.

Then, as women began to assert themselves in all phases of life, including the birth of their own children, a revolution in the business of "birthing babies" took place. Where once only doctors could tread, midwives began to ply their trade, in hospitals, birthing centers, and sometimes, even in the home. Women, perhaps for the first time in history, could choose how and under what circumstances they would give birth to their babies.

Midwives are health care professionals who are usually, but not always, licensed by the states to care for women during "normal" pregnancy, labor and childbirth. They are not permitted to perform Cesarean sections, handle pregnancies that are not "normal," such as where the mother has a health history which indicates that complications can be anticipated or where a dangerous condition has been diagnosed. Also, a midwife must work in association with a physician who must be available to the midwife's patients in times of need.

Many midwives are certified nurse midwives, who are R.N.s with a master's degree level of special training. There are also "lay" midwives, who are not nurses but who have received appropriate training in midwifery. Some states license lay midwives if they can pass a rigorous test; others do not. Non-licensed lay midwives may practice in some states but not in others. Check with your state Medical Licensing Board for the laws in your jurisdiction.

The whole point of midwives and natural childbirth, whether at home (allowed in some states), at a birthing center (a facility designed to accommodate mothers who desire unmedicated, noninterventionist childbirth) or a hospital, is to give the parents a more personal birth experience and as much control over the *normal* delivery as possible.

This experience can be patient power at its finest, as illustrated by Lora's story. Lora wanted natural childbirth but her doctor urged her to have "prepared childbirth," which would have included, among other things, an episiotomy (an incision from the vagina toward the anus), an enema, an internal fetal monitor and an external fetal monitor. (*Not that these are wrong. For many women, perhaps most women, they are not. They were just wrong for Lora.)* When she couldn't get the ob/gyn to change his mind about her delivery, Lora switched to the care of a certified nurse midwife who worked with a birthing center close to her home. Here, in her own words, is what Lora experienced:

"*I arrived at the birthing center at 5:30* A.M. *After walking around [they allow that at birthing centers] for awhile, I relaxed in the bedroom. The labor nurse kept me company along with my husband and the center owner. When the contractions became more intense, the certified nurse and midwife did some perineal massage and my husband rubbed my back. She told me to tell her if I had the urge to bear down. By 6:50 I did, so she swabbed down the area with a disinfectant and Ben was born at 6:53. No prep, enema, IV, episiotomy, fetal monitor, anesthesia or analgesics. No surgical garb, glaring lights or stirrups. My baby never left my side, except to be weighed. He went into the next room on his Daddy's bare chest, warmed in his arms. By noon (five hours after his birth) we all returned home. I have never experienced such a moment of intense joy as the birth of my son."*

Lora did it "her way" and the result was a joyful memory that she will carry with her for as long as she lives.

Midwives and natural childbirth are not for everybody. But if you think they may be for you, be sure that you check the training, credentials, experience and philosophy of the midwife before you retain his or her services. (Yes, there are a few male midwives. Or should I say, midhusbands?) Also, be sure to meet the ob/gyn he or she is associated with and check that doctor's credentials, since the physician is the one who will treat you in the event anything abnormal or potentially dangerous to the mother or child occurs. Finally, be sure to investigate the birthing facility as carefully as you would a hospital where you would have major surgery performed.

• Pharmacists •

Pharmacists should not be confused with entrepreneurs who run "drug stores" which dispense everything from diet pills to pantyhose. No, pharmacists are health care professionals who dispense drugs to patients as prescribed in writing by a physician. And while they may also be merchants who sell sunglasses and magazines, we will restrict our discussion to their professional function.

A pharmacist is a vital member of your health care team who provides you with several important services besides dispensing drugs for your prescribed medication dollar. (All right, for your prescribed medication *fifty* dollars.) These services are:

Acting as a fail-safe: Physicians sometimes make mistakes. Members of their staffs also make mistakes. Thus, throughout the health care system, fail-safe mechanisms have been established for the patient's protection. When it comes to drugs, that job falls upon the pharmacist.

This job is especially important today because so many of the drugs that are so very effective in treating us also have some potentially serious side effects. In addition, their therapeutic range (the amount in the blood stream that works effectively on the malady being treated) can be very narrow, so a big part of what a pharmacist does is to ensure that the medication has been prescribed in a proper dose and for the proper purpose. There is another potential problem: according to Dr. Sidney Wolfe and Ralph Nader's Health Research Group, doctors sometimes prescribe drugs which are ineffective for the malady they are supposed to treat. Your pharmacist may be able to catch this mistake before you ingest useless drugs.

Hint: Don't be offended if the pharmacist asks you what the prescription is for. He or she isn't being nosy. On the contrary, it is your pharmacist's business to know why you are taking the medicine so that he or she can effectively fulfill his or her fail-safe responsibility. If the pharmacist doesn't ask, make a point of telling him or her. Remember, doctors don't always put the reason for the medicine on the prescription.

Your pharmacist will also check to make sure the drug you are taking does not adversely react to other medications that may have been prescribed for you. Remember, the drugs that are used today are very potent. And, if you go to more than one doctor, each may not know what the other one has been prescribing. Thus, even though you may use more than one doctor, always use the same pharmacist to maximize your protection.

Hint: If you have more than one doctor, make sure each knows what the other one is doing to prevent treatments that may be at cross purposes with each other.

Providing information: Doctors don't always know as much about the drugs they prescribe as does the pharmacist who fills the doctor's prescription. That's because pharmacists have far more training in drugs and their effects than doctors and usually engage in continuing education about prescribed medications which may, in fact, exceed that of the doctor. Plus, doctors don't always do the best job informing their patients of all they need to know about dosage, potential side effects and whether the drug can impair the patient's ability to drive an automobile. The pharmacist has this information and should tell it to the patient even if the physician already has. After all, the doctor could have left something out. And besides, patients do forget.

Hint: If you are having a problem with a prescribed drug and are concerned, call your doctor. If he or she can't be reached, call your pharmacist.

Helping with over-the-counter medicines: There are many medicines that are sold without prescriptions. Some work very well. Others have little value except to the company which sells them to an unsuspecting public. Your pharmacist should be able to tell you which is which.

Hint: This is not the same thing as prescribing medications for you. If you have a health problem of any real concern, ask your doctor what to do about it, not your pharmacist.

Note:

There is a new trend taking place, in which doctors are dispensing the medications they prescribe. As you might expect, this has caused some controversy. On the plus side for patients is a reduction in the cost of the drugs, since the doctor can sell them for less due to the fact that the cost of overhead does not have to be included in the price. On the minus side, physicians who dispense their own drugs (other than giving away free starter samples which are given to them by drug salespersons) may find the financial incentive to write a prescription hard to resist, and the patient loses the benefits which a good pharmacist provides.

Christian Science Practitioners

I can hear you asking, "What in the world is he doing talking about religion in a book about doctors?" Well, I'll tell you. Christian Science is definitely a religion, but practitioners (as opposed to members) are also health care semi-professionals who keep regular office hours and charge for their healing services.

Christian Science practitioners cannot diagnose nor prescribe drugs nor provide any "traditional" medical service of any kind. They are, in fact, a spiritual ministry, but a ministry with a difference. That difference is this: Christian Science practitioners are accepted as an effective source of healing by many health insurance companies which will pay insurance benefits for the costs of a practitioner's "treatment." Medicare and other government health benefits may not, however, be used to pay for the services of a Christian Science practitioner since that would violate the First Amendment prohibition against state support of religion.

Practitioners are permitted to practice in all fifty states as an exercise of religion. To become a practitioner, a member of the Christian Science Church must be certified by the church, which is only done after proving the applicant's effectiveness in healing, high moral character and readiness to meet the tasks which face practitioners.

A list of all practitioners broken down by locale can be found each month in *The Christian Science Journal,* located in any Christian Science Reading Room.

• The Rest Of The Team •

There are, of course, many other health care professionals who serve millions of Americans every day. The following are just a few of them.

Psychologists: Psychologists are in the practice of understanding, predicting and influencing human behavior. Psychologists work in many different areas—from behavior modification to helping us solve difficulties in interpersonal relationships. Psychologists are Ph.D.s, and are permitted to hypnotize and to administer tests such as aptitude tests or tests which reveal personality characteristics. But they may not prescribe medications, diagnose medical conditions or engage in invasive procedures. Health insurance may or may not pay for their services.

Acupuncturists: Acupuncturists insert needles into the surface of the body (which supposedly doesn't hurt) to prevent pain, or to normalize physiological functions or correct certain dysfunctions of the body. The practice comes from the Orient, where they even use it in place of drug-induced anesthesia, something that is beginning to find acceptance in the West.

Physical Therapists: Physical therapists work with physicians to plan, organize and direct programs of care for persons who are in pain or disabled due to illness, accident or handicap. PTs can administer and interpret tests, but must stay in contact with the referring physician regarding the patient's progress.

Needless to say, there are many others. There are opticians, dentists, speech pathologists, nutritionists, audiologists, physician's assistants and many, many more—enough, in fact, to fill a whole book. (Hey, wait a minute! There's an idea! Now if I can just convince my editor. . .)

Notes To The Chart

As I have stated before, I cannot express my admiration for nurses and other nonphysician members of your health care team in strong enough terms (including x-ray technicians, dieticians, lab technicians, etc.). These professionals do the hands-on work of health care. Without them, doctors would be very limited as to what they could do and the number of patients they could treat. These dedicated professionals literally make it possible for doctors to do the job we have trained so hard to be able to do.

The section on pharmacists in this chapter is of vital concern to every patient who must take prescription drugs. Pharmacists *are* storehouses of useful and helpful information about everything from side effects to the proper storage of your medicine. In fact, I frequently consult with the clinical pharmacists in the hospitals where I am on staff in order to achieve "state-of-the-art" medical care for my patients. You should do the same with your local pharmacist. After all, you, your doctor and your pharmacist all have one common goal—your good health.

Supplement

There can be no patient power without access to accurate and understandable information. Happily, a lack of access to information is not one of the problems facing consumers of medical care in this country. Bookstores have racks and racks of books on almost every medical topic. Medical foundations and consumer groups are a veritable storehouse of information on specific maladies as well as general health care. The media features stories about health and medicine on almost a daily basis. And, of course, your doctor is there to answer or find the answer to virtually every medical question you may have.

The following is just a sample of the sources of information available to you. Some of these organizations also provide physician referral services and/or assistance in paying for medical treatment.

Note: Many of these organizations also have local or state chapters. Ask your doctor, or check your local phone directory.

AIDS NATIONAL HOTLINE:
1-800-342-AIDS (24 hours a day,
7 days a week)

AMERICAN ACADEMY OF FACIAL, PLASTIC & RECONSTRUCTIVE SURGERY
1101 Vermont Ave. NW—Suite 404
Washington, DC, 20005
(202) 842-4500 or 1-800-332-FACE

AMERICAN ACADEMY OF FAMILY PHYSICIANS
1740 West 92nd St.
Kansas City, MO 64114
(816) 333-9700

AMERICAN ACADEMY OF PEDIATRICS
1411 Northwest Point Blvd.
P.O. Box 927
Elk Grove Village, IL 60009-0927

AMERICAN BOARD OF INTERNAL MEDICINE
3624 Market St.
Philadelphia, PA 19104
(215) 243-1500

AMERICAN CANCER SOCIETY HOTLINE: 1-800-4-CANCER
National Headquarters
90 Park Ave.
New York, NY 10016

AMERICAN CHIROPRACTIC ASSOCIATION
1701 Clarendon Blvd.
Arlington, VA 22209
(703) 276-8800

AMERICAN COLLEGE OF SURGEONS
50 E. Erie St.
Chicago, IL 60611-2797
(Supplies list of F.A.C.S. Surgeons)

AMERICAN HEART ASSOCIATION
National Center
7320 Greenville Ave.
Dallas, TX 75231
(214) 706-1340

AMERICAN MEDICAL ASSOCIATION
535 N. Dearborn St.
Chicago, IL 60610
(312) 645-5000

ARTHRITIS FOUNDATION
National Office
1314 Spring St. NW
Atlanta, GA 30309

CANCER INFORMATION:
1-800-4-CANCER
(U.S. Dept. of Health & Human Services)

CENTERS FOR DISEASE CONTROL
1600 Clifton Rd. NE
Atlanta, GA 30333
(404) 329-3311

CONSUMERS FOR MEDICAL QUALITY, INC.
P.O. Box 1052
Merced, CA 95341
(209) 723-3505

CYSTIC FIBROSIS ASSOCIATION
6000 Executive Blvd.—Suite 510
Rockville, MD 20852
(301) 881-9130

EPILEPSY FOUNDATION OF AMERICA
4351 Garden City Dr.
Landover, MD 20785
(301) 459-3700

FDA DRUG HOTLINE: 1-800-336-4797

FAMILY SERVICE OF AMERICA
4700 W. Lake Park Dr.
Milwaukee, WI 53224
(414) 359-2111

HEALTH & HUMAN SERVICE HOTLINE:
(301) 962-3396
P.O. Box 17303
Baltimore, MD 21203-7303

MAYO CLINIC FOUNDATION
Rochester, MN 55905
(507) 284-2511 or Mayo Clinic
(507) 284-4587

MEDIC ALERT FOUNDATION INTERNATIONAL
P.O. Box 1009
Turlock, CA 95381-1009
(209) 668-3333 or 1-800-ID ALERT

MEDICARE HOTLINE: 1-800-368-5779
(Re: improper bill or service)

MUSCULAR DYSTROPHY ASSOCIATION
810 Seventh Ave.
New York, NY 10019
(212) 586-0808

NATIONAL EASTER SEAL SOCIETY
2023 W. Ogden Ave.
Chicago, IL 60612
(312) 243-8400

NATIONAL FOUNDATION FOR ASTHMA, INC.
P.O. Box 30069
Tucson, AZ 85751-0069
(602) 323-6046

NATIONAL HEMOPHILIAC FOUNDATION
19 W. 34th St.–Suite 1204
New York, NY 10011
(212) 563-0211

NATIONAL HOSPICE ORGANIZATION
1901 N. Fort Meyer Dr.–Suite 307
Arlington, VA 22209
(703) 243-5900
(Maintains list of all hospices in the U.S.
—public referral service)

NATIONAL KIDNEY FOUNDATION
2 Park Ave.
New York, NY 10016
(212) 889-2210

NATIONAL MULTIPLE SCLEROSIS SOCIETY
205 E. 42nd Ave.
New York, NY 10017
(212) 986-3240

PEOPLE'S MEDICAL SOCIETY
14 E. Minor St.
Emmaus, PA 18049
(215) 967-2136

PUBLIC CITIZEN
Health Research Group
2000 P St. NW
Washington, DC 20036
(202) 872-0320

THE FIRST CHURCH OF CHRIST SCIENTIST
Christian Science Center
Boston, MA 02115

UNITED CEREBRAL PALSY ASSOCIATIONS, INC.
66 E. 34th St.
New York, NY 10016
(212) 481-6300

UNITED WAY
701 N. Fairfax St.
Alexandria, VA 22314
(703) 836-7100

VETERANS ADMINISTRATION
Washington, DC 20420

• Suggested Reading List •

There are many books on health and health care on the market today. Some are more p.r. than substance, especially some fad diet books, like "*The Pumpkin Pie Diet.*" Be sure to check with your physician before accepting the medical advice given in any book.

AMA Family Medical Guide (Random House)

Anatomy of an Illness (Bantam)

The American Cancer Society Cancer Book (Doubleday)

The Birth Center—An Approach to the Birth Experience (Prentice Hall)

Complete Guide to Prescription & Non Prescription Drugs (HP Books)

Complete Guide to Symptoms, Illness & Surgery (HP Books)

Good Housekeeping Family Health & Medical Guide (Hearst Books)

Life Wish by Paula M. Carroll (Medical Consumers Publishing Co.) One woman's horror story of medical malpractice.

Pills That Don't Work (Public Citizen Health Research Group)

Take This Book to the Hospital with You (Rodale Press)

• State Medical Licensing Boards •

If you wish to report your doctor to state authorities for unprofessional conduct, or if you have questions about your doctor's conduct, contact the following agency in your state:

ALABAMA STATE BOARD OF MEDICAL EXAMINERS
Executive Director
P.O. Box 946
Montgomery, AL 36102-0946
(205) 261-4116

ALASKA BOARD OF MEDICAL EXAMINERS
Div. of Occupational Licensing
Investigative Section
P.O. Box D
Juneau, AL 99811
(907) 465-2541

ARIZONA STATE BOARD OF MEDICAL EXAMINERS
Executive Director
1990 W. Camelback Rd. #401
Phoenix, AZ 85015
(602) 255-3751

ARKANSAS STATE MEDICAL BOARD
P.O. Box 102
Harrisburg, AR 72432-0102
(501) 578-2448

CALIFORNIA BOARD OF MEDICAL QUALITY ASSURANCE
Executive Director
1430 Howe Ave.
Sacramento, CA 95825
(916) 920-6393

COLORADO BOARD OF MEDICAL EXAMINERS
Program Administrator
132 State Services Building
1525 Sherman St.
Denver, CO 80203
(303) 866-2468

CONNECTICUT MEDICAL EXAMINING BOARD
Director
Div. of Medical Quality Assurance
150 Washington St.
Hartford, CT 06106
(203) 566-1482

DELAWARE STATE BOARD OF MEDICAL EXAMINERS
c/o Administrative Assistant
O'Neill Bldg.
P.O. Box 1401
Dover, DE 19903
(302) 736-4522

DISTRICT OF COLUMBIA COMMISSION ON LICENSURE TO PRACTICE THE HEALING ARTS
President
605 G St., NW—Room 202, Lower Level
Washington, DC 20001
(202) 727-9794

FLORIDA BOARD OF MEDICAL EXAMINERS
Executive Director
130 N. Monroe St.
Tallahassee, FL 32301
(904) 488-0595

GEORGIA COMPOSITE BOARD OF MEDICAL EXAMINERS
Executive Director
166 Pryor St. SW
Atlanta, GA 30303
(404) 656-3913 or -7067

HAWAII BOARD OF MEDICAL EXAMINERS
Executive Secretary
Dept. of Commerce & Consumer Affrs.
P.O. Box 3469
Honolulu, HI 96801
(808) 548-4392

IDAHO STATE BOARD OF MEDICINE
Executive Director
650 W. State St.
Boise, ID 83720
(208) 334-2822

ILLINOIS DEPARTMENT OF REGISTRATION AND EDUCATION
Director
320 W. Washington St.
Springfield, IL 62786
(217) 785-0820

also

State of Illinois Center
100 W. Randolph St. #9-300
Chicago, IL 60601
(312) 917-4500

INDIANA HEALTH PROFESSIONS SERVICE BUREAU
Executive Director
964 N. Pennsylvania
Indianapolis, IN 46204
(317) 232-2960

IOWA STATE BOARD OF MEDICAL EXAMINERS
Executive Director
1209 E. Court Ave.
Des Moines, IA 50319
(515) 281-6493 or -5171

KANSAS STATE BOARD OF HEALING ARTS
President
503 Kansas Ave. #500
Topeka, KS 66603-3449
(913) 296-7413

KENTUCKY STATE BOARD OF MEDICAL LICENSURE
Executive Director
Mall Office Center
400 Sherburn Ln.—Suite 222
Louisville, KY 40207
(502) 896-1516

LOUISIANA STATE BOARD OF MEDICAL EXAMINERS
President
830 Union St.
New Orleans, LA 70112
(504) 524-6763

MAINE BOARD OF REGISTRATION IN MEDICINE
Executive Secretary
Eastside Professional Building
RFD #3, Box 461
Waterville, ME 04901
(207) 873-2184

MARYLAND BOARD OF MEDICAL EXAMINERS
Executive Director
201 W. Preston St.
Baltimore, MD 21201
(301) 225-5900

MASSACHUSETTS BOARD OF REGISTRATION IN MEDICINE
Executive Director
100 Cambridge—Room 1507
Boston, MA 02202
(617) 727-3086 or -3087

MICHIGAN BOARD OF MEDICINE
Licensing Executive
P.O. Box 30018
611 W. Ottawa St.
Lansing, MI 48909
(517) 373-0680

MINNESOTA BOARD OF MEDICAL EXAMINERS
Executive Director
2700 University Ave. W.–Suite 106
St. Paul, MN 55114-1080
(612) 642-0538

MISSISSIPPI STATE BOARD OF MEDICAL LICENSURE
Executive Officer
2688-D Insurance Center Dr.
Jackson, MS 39216
(601) 354-6645

MISSOURI STATE BOARD OF REGISTRATION FOR THE HEALING ARTS
Executive Secretary
P.O. Box 4
Jefferson City, MO 65102
(314) 751-2334 Ext. 151

MONTANA BOARD OF MEDICAL EXAMINERS
Administrative Assistant
1424 9th Ave.
Helena, MT 59620-0407
(406) 444-4284

NEBRASKA STATE BOARD OF EXAMINERS IN MEDICINE & SURGERY
Executive Secretary
P.O. Box 95007
Lincoln, NB 68509
(402) 471-2115

NEVADA STATE BOARD OF MEDICAL EXAMINERS
Executive Secretary
1281 Terminal Way–Suite 213
P.O. Box 7238
Reno, NV 89510
(702) 329-2559

NEW HAMPSHIRE BOARD OF REGISTRATION IN MEDICINE
Executive Secretary
Health & Welfare Bldg.
Hazen Dr.
Concord, NH 03301
(603) 271-4501

NEW JERSEY STATE BOARD OF MEDICAL EXAMINERS
Executive Secretary
28 W. State St.–Room 914
Trenton, NJ 08608
(609) 292-4843

NEW MEXICO STATE BOARD OF MEDICAL EXAMINERS
Bureau Chief
Bataan Mem. Bldg. 3rd Floor
P.O. Drawer 1388
Sante Fe, NM 87504-1388
(505) 827-9934

NEW YORK STATE BOARD FOR MEDICINE
Executive Secretary
Cultural Education Center–Room 3023
Empire State Plaza
Albany, NY 12230
(518) 474-3841

NORTH CAROLINA BOARD OF MEDICAL EXAMINERS
Executive Secretary
222 N. Person St. #214
Raleigh, NC 27601
(919) 833-5321

NORTH DAKOTA STATE BOARD OF MEDICAL EXAMINERS
Executive Secretary
City Center Plaza
418 E. Broadway #C-10
Bismarck, ND 58501
(701) 223-9485

OHIO STATE MEDICAL BOARD
Executive Director
65 S. Front St. #510
Columbus, OH 43266-0315
(614) 466-3938

OKLAHOMA BOARD OF MEDICAL EXAMINERS
Administrator
P.O. Box 18256
Oklahoma City, OK 73154
(405) 848-6841

OREGON BOARD OF MEDICAL EXAMINERS
Executive Secretary
1002 Loyalty Bldg.
317 SW Alder St.
Portland, OR 97204
(503) 229-5770

PENNSYLVANIA STATE BOARD OF MEDICAL EDUCATION & LICENSURE
Administrative Asst.
P.O. Box 2649
Harrisburg, PA 17105-2649
(717) 787-2381

RHODE ISLAND BOARD OF MEDICAL REVIEW
Executive Director
100 India St.
Providence, RI 02903
(401) 227-3855 or -2507

SOUTH CAROLINA STATE BOARD OF MEDICAL EXAMINERS
Executive Director
1315 Blanding St.
Columbia, SC 29201
(803) 758-3361

SOUTH DAKOTA STATE BOARD OF MEDICAL & OSTEOPATHIC EXAMINERS
Executive Secretary
608 West Ave. No.
Sioux Falls, SD 57104
(605) 336-1965

TENNESSEE STATE BOARD OF MEDICAL EXAMINERS
Reg. Board Administrator
283 Plus Park Blvd.
Nashville, TN 37219-5407
(615) 367-6200

TEXAS STATE BOARD OF MEDICAL EXAMINERS
Executive Director
P.O. Box 13562
Capitol Station
Austin, TX 78711
(512) 452-1078

UTAH PHYSICIANS LICENSING BOARD
Director Div. of Occupational & Professional Licensing
160 East 300 South
P.O. Box 45802
Salt Lake City, UT 84145
(801) 530-6628

VERMONT BOARD OF MEDICAL PRACTICE
Executive Director
Licensing & Registration
Redstone Building
26 Terrace St.
Montpelier, VT 05602
(802) 828-2363

VIRGINIA STATE BOARD OF MEDICINE
Executive Director
1601 Rolling Hills Dr.
Richmond, VA 23229-5005
(804) 662-9900

WASHINGTON DEPARTMENT OF PROFESSIONAL LICENSING
Executive Secretary
Medical Board
P.O. Box 9649
Olympia, WA 98504
(206) 753-3779

WEST VIRGINIA BOARD OF MEDICINE
Executive Director
100 Dee Dr. #104
Charleston, WV 25311
(304) 348-2921

WISCONSIN DEPARTMENT OF REGISTRATION AND LICENSING
Administrative Assistant
P.O. Box 8935
Madison, WI 53708
(608) 266-2811

WYOMING BOARD OF MEDICAL EXAMINERS
Executive Secretary
Hathaway Building 4th Floor
Cheyenne, WY 82002
(307) 777-6463

GUAM BOARD OF MEDICAL EXAMINERS
Administrator
Dept. of Public Health & Social Services
P.O. Box 2816
Agana, Guam 96910
(671) 734-2783

VIRGIN ISLANDS BOARD OF MEDICAL EXAMINERS
Secretary
St. Thomas Hosp., Dept. of Health
P.O. Box 7309
St. Thomas, Virgin Islands 00801
(809) 776-6311

Index

R

S

T

U

V

X